G. Burg ■ W. Kempf (Eds.)

Cutaneous Lymphomas: Unusual Cases 2

G. BURG W. KEMPF (EDS.)

Cutaneous Lymphomas
Unusual Cases 2

Co-Editors
S. MICHAELIS and J. FEIT

Technical Assistance
B. FRUET and PH. COLLING

WITH 236 COLOUR FIGURES

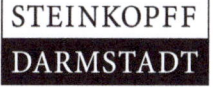

STEINKOPFF
DARMSTADT

GÜNTER BURG, MD
Professor of Dermatology and Venerology
Department of Dermatology
University Hospital of Zürich
Gloriastrasse 31
8091 Zürich, Switzerland

WERNER KEMPF, MD
Department of Dermatology
University Hospital of Zürich
Gloriastrasse 31
8091 Zürich, Switzerland

ISBN 978-3-7985-9999-4
Steinkopff Verlag Darmstadt

Cataloging-in-Publication Data applied for
A catalog record for this book is available from the Library of Congress. Bibliographic information published
by Die Deutsche Bibliothek. Die Deutsche Bibliothek lists this publication in the Deutsche Nationalbibliografie:
detailed bibliographic data is available in the Internet at <http://dnb.ddb.de>.

Steinkopff Verlag Darmstadt is a part of Springer Science+Business Media

© Steinkopff Verlag Darmstadt 2006
Softcover reprint of the hardcover 1st edition 2006

Production: Klemens Schwind
Cover-Design: Erich Kirchner, Heidelberg
Typesetting: K + V Fotosatz GmbH, Beerfelden
Printing and binding: Stürtz GmbH, Würzburg

SPIN 11662808   105/7231-5 4 3 2 1 0 – Printed on acid-free paper

Preface

The elaboration of the WHO/EORTC-Classification for cutaneous lymphomas (G. Burg, E.S. Jaffe, W. Kempf et al. in Pathology & Genetics of Skin Tumours, World Health Organisation Classification of Tumours. E. LeBoit, G. Burg, D. Weedon, A. Sarasin (Eds.). IARC Press Lyon, 2006. ISBN 9283224140) is a milestone in the long lasting process of finding a consensus in the nomenclature for nodal and cutaneous lymphoproliferative disorders. Despite the widespread acceptance of the WHO/EORTC-Classification, there are still cases which do not fit into the framework and thus offer even greater diagnostic challenges.

This book, like the first volume on unusual cases of cutaneous lymphomas, again presents a number of such fascinating cases, showing distinct features of mature T-cell and NK-cell neoplasms, mature B-cell neoplasms and immature haematopoietic malignancies.

The descriptions are given by experienced dermatologists and pathologists. Each chapter contains a short comment, excellent clinical and histopathologic illustrations, and carefully selected references. Looking through these cases may help the reader to then recognize other similar cases of rare cutaneous lymphomas which might be included into the WHO/EORTC-Classification as new distinct entities in the future.

Zürich, February 2006

GÜNTER BURG
WERNER KEMPF

Table of Contents

3 Immature Hematopoietic Malignancies

■ Addresses

ABBOTT JARED J., MD, PhD
Resident in Pathology
Mayo Clinic
Department of Dermatology
Dermatopathology Division
200 First ST SW
Rochester, Minnesota 55905, USA
abbott.jared@mayo.edu

AHMED IFTIKHAR, MD
Mayo Clinic
Department of Dermatology
Dermatopathology Division
200 First ST SW
Rochester, Minnesota 55905, USA
ahmed.iftikhar2@mayo.edu

ASAGOE KENJI, MD
Okayama University
Graduate School of Medicine
and Dentistry
Department of Dermatology
2-5-1 Shikata-cho
Okayama 700-8558, Japan
asakoshi@cc.okayama-u.ac.jp

BAGOT MARTINE, MD, PhD
Professor of Dermatology
and Venerology
Hôpital Henri Mondor
Department of Dermatology
51 Avenue de Lattre de Tassigny
94010 Créteil Cedex, France
martine.bagot@hmn.aphp.fr

BEKKENK MARCEL W., MD
Leiden University Medical Center
Department of Dermatology
Albinusdreef 2
2333 ZA Leiden, Netherlands
M.W.Bekkenk@lumc.nl

BELOUSOVA IRENA E., MD, PhD
Medical Military Academy
Department of Dermatology
Lebedeva str. 6
Saint-Petersburg, 194044, Russia
beloussova@yahoo.com

BERNENGO MARIA GRAZIA, MD
Professor of Dermatology
and Venereology
University of Turin
Department of Biomedical Sciences
and Human Oncology
Section of Dermatology
Via Cherasco 23
10126 Torino, Italy
mariagrazia.bernengo@unito.it

BOUDOVA LUDMILA, MD, PhD
Charles University
Medical Faculty Hospital
Sikl's Department of Pathology
Alej Svobody 80
30460 Pilsen, Czech Republic
boudova@medima.cz

BURG GÜNTER, MD
Professor of Dermatology
and Venereology
University Hospital of Zürich
Department of Dermatology
Gloriastrasse 31
8091 Zürich, Switzerland
burg@derm.unizh.ch

CERRONI LORENZO, MD
Universitätsklinik für Dermatologie
und Venerologie Graz
Auenbruggerplatz 8
8036 Graz, Austria
lorenzo.cerroni@meduni-graz.at

CHIMENTI SERGIO, MD
Chairman and Professor
University of Rome Tor Vergata
Department of Dermatology
PTV – Policlinico di Tor Vergata
V. le Oxford 81
00133 Rome, Italy
chimenti@dermatologica.it

CHRISTEN B., MD
Stadtspital Triemli
Department of Ophthalmology
Birmensdorferstrasse 497
8063 Zürich, Switzerland
elmar.messmer@triemli.stzh.ch

CITARELLA LUIGI, MD
Resident in Dermatology
University of Rome Tor Vergata
Department of Dermatology
PTV – Policlinico di Tor Vergata
V. le Oxford 81
00133 Rome, Italy
l.citarella@libero.it

DRÉNO BRIGITTE, MD
University of Skin Oncology
Hotel Dieu
Place Alexis Ricordeau
44093 Nantes Cedex 01, France
brigitte.dreno@wanadoo.fr

DUMMER REINHARD, MD
Professor of Dermatology
and Venereology
University Hospital of Zürich
Department of Dermatology
Gloriastrasse 31
8091 Zürich, Switzerland
reinhard.dummer@usz.ch

FEITH JOSEF, MD
Medical Faculty of Masaryk University
2nd Institute of Pathology
Jihlavská 20
620 00 Brno, Czech Republic
jfeit@ics.muni.cz

FRUET BARBARA
Technical Assistant
University Hospital of Zürich
Department of Dermatology
Gloriastrasse 31
8091 Zürich, Switzerland
barbara.fruet@usz.ch

GIBSON LAWRENCE E., MD
Professor of Dermatology
Mayo Clinic
Mayo School of Medicine
Department of Dermatology
Dermatopathology Division
200 First ST SW
Rochester, Minnesota 55905, USA
gibson.lawrence@mayo.edu

GOLLING PHILIPPA, MD
Dermatologist
University Hospital of Zürich
Department of Dermatology
Gloriastrasse 31
8091 Zürich, Switzerland
philippa.golling@usz.ch

HARRIS ROLAND M., MD, MBA
Assistant Professor of Dermatology
and Pathology
University of Utah
Department of Dermatology
School of Medicine, 4B454
30 North 1900 East
Salt Lake City, Utah 84132, USA

HASHIZUME HIDEO, MD
Associate Professor
Hamamatsu University
School of Medicine
Department of Dermatology
1-20-1 Handa-yama
Hamamatsu 431-3192, Japan
hihashiz@hama-med.ac.jp

HES O., MD
Charles University
Medical Faculty Hospital
Sikl's Department of Pathology
Alej Svobody 80
30460 Pilsen, Czech Republic
hes@medima.cz

HEULE FREERK, MD, PhD
Erasmus MC University
Medical Center Rotterdam
Department of Dermatology
Room Sv. 221
Dr. Molewaterplein 40
3015 GE Rotterdam, Netherlands
f.heule.1@erasmusmc.nl

HINSHAW MOLLY A., MD
Assistant Professor of Dermatology
University of Wisconsin
Department of Dermatology
One South Park Street, 7th Floor
Madison, WI 53715, USA
mhinshaw4@hotmail.com

HOEFNAGEL JULIETTE, MD
Leiden University Medical Center
Department of Dermatology
Albinusdreef 2
2333 ZA Leiden, Netherlands
j.hoefnagel@lumc.nl

HORIBE TAKAHIRO, MD
Instructor of Dermatology
Hamamatsu University
School of Medicine
Department of Dermatology
1-20-1 Handa-yama
Hamamatsu 431-3192, Japan
horibe22@hama-med.ac.jp

IWATSUKI KEIJI, MD, PhD
Professor of Dermatology
Okayama University
Graduate School
of Medicine and Dentistry
Department of Dermatology
2-5-1 Shikata-cho
Okayama 700-8558, Japan
keijiiwa@cc.okayama-u.ac.jp

JANSSEN PATTY M. ,MD
Leiden University Medical Center
Department of Dermatology
Albinusdreef 2
2333 ZA Leiden, Netherlands
p.m.jansen@lumc.nl

JESKANEN LEILA, MD
Specialist in Dermatology
and Venereology
Specialist in Pathology
Helsinki University
Central Hospital
Skin and Allergy Hospital
Laboratory Division (HUSLAB)
Skin pathology laboratory
PL 160
00029 HUS Helsinki Finland
leila.jeskanen@hus.fi

KARENKO LEENA, MD, PhD
Researcher
University of Helsinki
Department of Dermatology
Meilahdentie 2
00250 Helsinki Finland
leena.p.karenkoi@hus.fi

KAZAKOV DMITRY V., MD, PhD
Charles University
Medical Faculty Hospital
Sikl's Department of Pathology
Alej Svobody 80
30460 Pilsen, Czech Republic
kazakov@medima.cz

KEMPF WERNER, MD
Specialist in Dermatology
and Venereology
University Hospital of Zürich
Department of Dermatology
Gloriastrasse 31
8091 Zürich, Switzerland
kempf@derm.unizh.ch

KERL HELMUT, MD
Professor of Dermatology
and Venereology
Universitätsklinik für Dermatologie
und Venerologie Graz
Auenbruggerplatz 8
8036 Graz, Austria
helmut.kerl@meduni-graz.at

KUNTSCHER V., MD
Charles University
Medical Faculty Hospital
Sikl's Department of Pathology
Alej Svobody 80
304 60 Pilsen, Czech Republic
kuntscher@fnPlzen.cz

LAETSCH BARBARA, MD
University Hospital of Zürich
Department of Dermatology
Gloriastrasse 31
8091 Zürich, Switzerland
barbara.laetsch@usz.ch

LANGERAK ANTON W., MD
Erasmus MC University
Medical Center Rotterdam
Department of Immunology
P.O. Box 1738
3000 DR Rotterdam, Netherlands
a.langerak@erasmusmc.nl

LONGLEY B. JACK, MD
Professor of Dermatology
University of Wisconsin
Department of Dermatology
One South Park Street, 7th Floor
Madison, WI 53715, USA
bjlongley@dermatology.wisc.edu

MATSUURA HIRONORI, MD
Okayama University
Graduate School of Medicine
and Dentistry
Department of Dermatology
2-5-1 Shikata-cho
Okayama 700-8558, Japan
hiromatu@cc.okayama-u.ac.jp

MEIJER CHRIS J.L.M., MD
Professor of Pathology
Vrije Universiteit Medical Center
Department of Pathology
De Boelelaan 1117
1816 TH Amsterdam, Netherlands
cjlm.meijer@azvu.nl

MESSMER ELMAR, MD
Professor
Stadtspital Triemli
Department of Ophthalmology
Birmensdorferstrasse 497
8063 Zürich, Switzerland
elmar.messmer@triemli.stzh.ch

MICHAELIS SONJA, MD
Assistant Doctor
University Hospital of Zürich
Department of Dermatology
Gloriastrasse 31
8091 Zürich, Switzerland
sonja.michaelis@usz.ch

MICHAL MICHAL, MD
Charles University
Medical Faculty Hospital
Sikl's Department of Pathology
Alej Svobody 80
30460 Pilsen, Czech Republic
michal@medima.cz

MIDDELDORP JAAP M., MD, PhD
Professor of Pathology
VU University Medical Center
Department of Pathology
P. O. Box 7057
1007 MB Amsterdam, Netherlands
j.middeldorp@vumc.nl

MORIZANE SHIN, MD
Okayama University
Graduate School of Medicine
and Dentistry
Department of Dermatology
2-5-1 Shikata-cho
Okayama 700-8558, Japan

MUKENŠNABL P., MD
Charles University
Medical Faculty Hospital
Sikl's Department of Pathology
Alej Svobody 80
30460 Pilsen, Czech Republic
mukensnabl@medima.cz

MUTASIM DIYA F., MD
Professor and Chairman
University of Cincinnati
College of Medicine
Department of Dermatology
231 Albert Sabin Way, Room 7409
Cincinnati, OH 45267-0592, USA
diya.mutasim@uc.edu

NOVELLI MAURO, PhD
University of Turin
Department of Biomedical Sciences
and Human Oncology
Section of Dermatology
Via Cherasco 23
10126 Torino, Italy
mauro.novelli@unito.it

OHTSUKA MIKIO, MD, PhD
Fukushima Medical University
School of Medicine
Department of Dermatology
1-Hikariga-oka
Fukushima 960-1295, Japan
motsuka@fmu.ac.jp

OONO TAKASHI, MD
Okayama University
Graduate School of Medicine
and Dentistry
Department of Dermatology
2-5-1 Shikata-cho
Okayama 700-8558, Japan
otakashi@cc.okayama-u.ac.jp

PITTELKOW MARK R., MD
Professor of Dermatology
Mayo Clinic
Department of Dermatology
Dermatopathology Division
200 First ST SW
Rochester, Minnesota, 55905, USA
pittelkow.mark@mayo.edu

QUAGLINO PIETRO, MD, PhD
University of Turin
Department of Biomedical Sciences
and Human Oncology
Section of Dermatology
Via Cherasco 23
10126 Torino, Italy
pietro.quaglino@unito.it

QUEREUX GAELLE, MD
University of Skin Oncology
Hotel Dieu
Place Alexis Ricordeau
44093 Nantes Cedex 01, France
gaelle.quereux@chu-nantes.fr

RANKI ANNAMARI, MD, PhD
Professor of Dermatology
and Venereology
Helsinki University Hospital
Department of Dermatology
P.O. Box 160
00029 HUS Helsinki, Finland
annamari.ranki@hus.fi

SALE TANYA, MD
Dermatology Resident
University of Wisconsin
Department of Dermatology
One South Park Street, 7th Floor
Madison, WI 53715, USA
tanyasale@yahoo.com

SAMOLITIS NANCY J., MD
Resident in Dermatology
University of Utah
Department of Dermatology
School of Medicine, 4B454
30 North 1900 East
Salt Lake City, Utah 84132, USA
nancysamolitis@yahoo.com

Sandberg Yorick, MD
Erasmus MC University
Medical Center Rotterdam
Department of Immunology
Dr. Molewaterplein 50
3015 GE Rotterdam, Netherlands
y.sandberg@erasmusmc.nl

Schaerer Leo, MD
University Hospital of Zürich
Department of Dermatology
Gloriastrasse 31
8091 Zürich, Switzerland
leo.schaerer@usz.ch

Sekulic Aleksandar, MD, PhD
Resident in Dermatology
Mayo Clinic
Department of Dermatology
Dermatopathology Division
200 First ST SW
Rochester, Minnesota 55905, USA
sekulic.aleksandar@mayo.edu

Stevens Servi, J. C., PhD
Researcher
VU University Medical Center
Department of Pathology
P.O.Box 7057
1007 MB Amsterdam, Netherlands
s.stevens@vumc.nl

Takigawa Masahiro, MD
Professor of Dermatology
Hamamatsu University
School of Medicine
Department of Dermatology
1-20-1 Handa-yama
Hamamatsu 431-3192, Japan
takigawa@hama-med.ac.jp

Tomita Kouichi, MD
Chief in Dermatology
Shizuoka City Shizuoka Hospital
Department of Dermatology
10-93 Outemachi
Shizuoka 420-8630, Japan
kinjohtenka@yahoo.co.jp

Twersky Joy M., MD
University Dermatology Center
2525 W. University Ave., Suite 402
Muncie, Indiana 47303, USA
jtwersky@udcin.com

Vermeer Maarten H., MD, PhD
Dermatologist
Leiden University Medical Center
Department of Dermatology
Albinusdreef 2
2333 ZA Leiden, Netherlands
m.h.vermeer@lumc.nl

Wechsler Janine, MD
Hôpital Henri Mondor
Department of Pathology
51 Avenue de Lattre de Tassigny
94010 Créteil Cedex, France
janine.wechsler@hmn.ap-hop-paris.fr

Weenig Roger H., MD, MhD
Assistant Professor of Dermatology
Mayo Clinic
Department of Dermatology
Dermatopathology Division
200 First ST SW
Rochester, Minnesota 55905, USA
weenig.roger@mayo.edu

Willemze Rein, MD
Professor of Dermatology
and Venereology
Leiden University Medical Center
Department of Dermatology
Albinusdreef 2
2333 ZA Leiden, Netherlands
willemze.dermatology@lumc.nl

Wood Gary S., MD
Johnson Professor and Chairman
University of Wisconsin
Department of Dermatology
One South Park Street, 7th Floor
Madison, WI 53715, USA
gwood@dermatology.wisc.edu

Yagi Hiroaki, MD
Assistant Professor of Dermatology
Hamamatsu University
School of Medicine
Department of Dermatology
1-20-1 Handa-yama
Hamamatsu 431-3192, Japan
hiroyagi@hama-med.ac.jp

1 Mature T-cell and NK-cell Neoplasms

Familial mycosis fungoides; involving a father and daughter

H. HORIBE, H. YAGI, M. TAKIGAWA and K. TOMITA

Age: 23 years (father), 28 years (daughter)
Sex: M (father), F (daughter)

Clinical features: A 27-year old girl presented with a 10-year history of wide spread erythematous plaques in 1999. Biopsy of the skin lesions showed a dense infiltrate of lymphoid cells in the upper dermis with epidermotropism. The most of these cells were CD3+CD4+CD7−CD45RO+CD30−CD56−CLA−. She was diagnosed as having mycosis fungoides, stage Ib, at that time. Her father was admitted to another hospital with mycosis fungoides, stage IVa, in 1999. His erythematous lesions and inguinal lymph nodes swelling appeared more than 6 months and 4 months before his admission, respectively. Skin biopsies showed a moderate infiltrate of large atypical lymphocytes into upper dermis with epidermotropism. There was no consanguineous marriage. Repeated serological tests for human T cell lymphotrophic virus type-I antibodies and EB virus infection were normal in both cases. The Southern blotting analyses of DNA from lesional skins revealed rearranged, non-germline bands in them with the use of a DNA probe ($C\beta_1$). The populations of these two lymphomas thought to be different, because the positions of non-germline bands were not identical.

Diagnosis: mycosis fungides involving a father and daughter.

Follow-up: Daughter: Initial treatment with PUVA and recombinant interferon-γ was ineffective. Skin electron beam irradiation (total dose, 40 Gy) resulted in partial improvement of the skin lesions. Four months after radiotherapy, however, she developed multiple skin tumors and marked lymphadenopathy. She was treated with a combination of biweekly CHOP, etoposide and methotrexate, which temporarily alleviated the condition. During the next 6 months, both the skin lesion and lymphadenopathy had progressed with the appearance of lymphoblasts in the bone marrow and peripheral blood. She died in 2001 of multiple organ failure at the age of 30 years.

Father: His skin lesions were resistant to topical corticosteroids. PUVA and low dose methotrexate temporarily alleviated the skin condition. Four years after the diagnosis of stage IVa, multiple skin tumors (Fig 3b) and a marked lymphadenopathy appeared. The treatments including chemotherapies and autologous peripheral blood stem cell transplantation were in vain. He died in 2004 of pulmonary alveolus hemorrhage at the age of 55 years.

Comment: Familial mycosis fungoides is extremely rare. Baykal C et al. reported their case and reviewed six familial cases. Onsets of the disease in three (25%) out of 12 patients (six families) including our cases were before 30 years of age. The young onset of the disease might be a characteristic feature of familial cases, because Burns et al. reported only 3.7% of patients develop mycosis fungoides before 30 years of age in their series of 246 patients. However, was not fully ruled out in some familial cases reported earlier. Our case showed three interesting features; 1) onset of the disease in the child preceded the parent, 2) the disease in two generations nearly simultaneously progressed to the terminal stage and 3) both showed resistance to chemotherapies and followed almost the same aggressive clinical course. Although not apparent, the existence of genetic or pathogenic elements in the cause of the disease was strongly suggested, in our case.

- **Fig. 1:** The daughter had erythematous plaques and multiple tumors (in 2000).
- **Fig. 2:** Histology of the daughter showed dense infiltrates of large lymphoid cells (a) forming Pautrier's, microabscesses (b).
- **Fig. 3:** The father initially had wide spread erythematous plaques (a; in 1999) and multiple tumors were developed later (b; in 2003).
- **Fig. 4:** Histology of the father showed upper dermal large lymphoid cell infiltrate.
- **Fig. 5:** Lymphoblasts in the bone marrow.

References

Baykal C, Buyukbabani N, Kaymaz R (2002) Familial mycosis fungoides. Br J Dermatol 146(6):1108–1110

Burns M, Ellis C, Cooper K et al. (1992) Mycosis Fungoides-type cutaneous T-cell lymphoma arising before 30 years of age. J Am Acad Dermatol 27:974–978

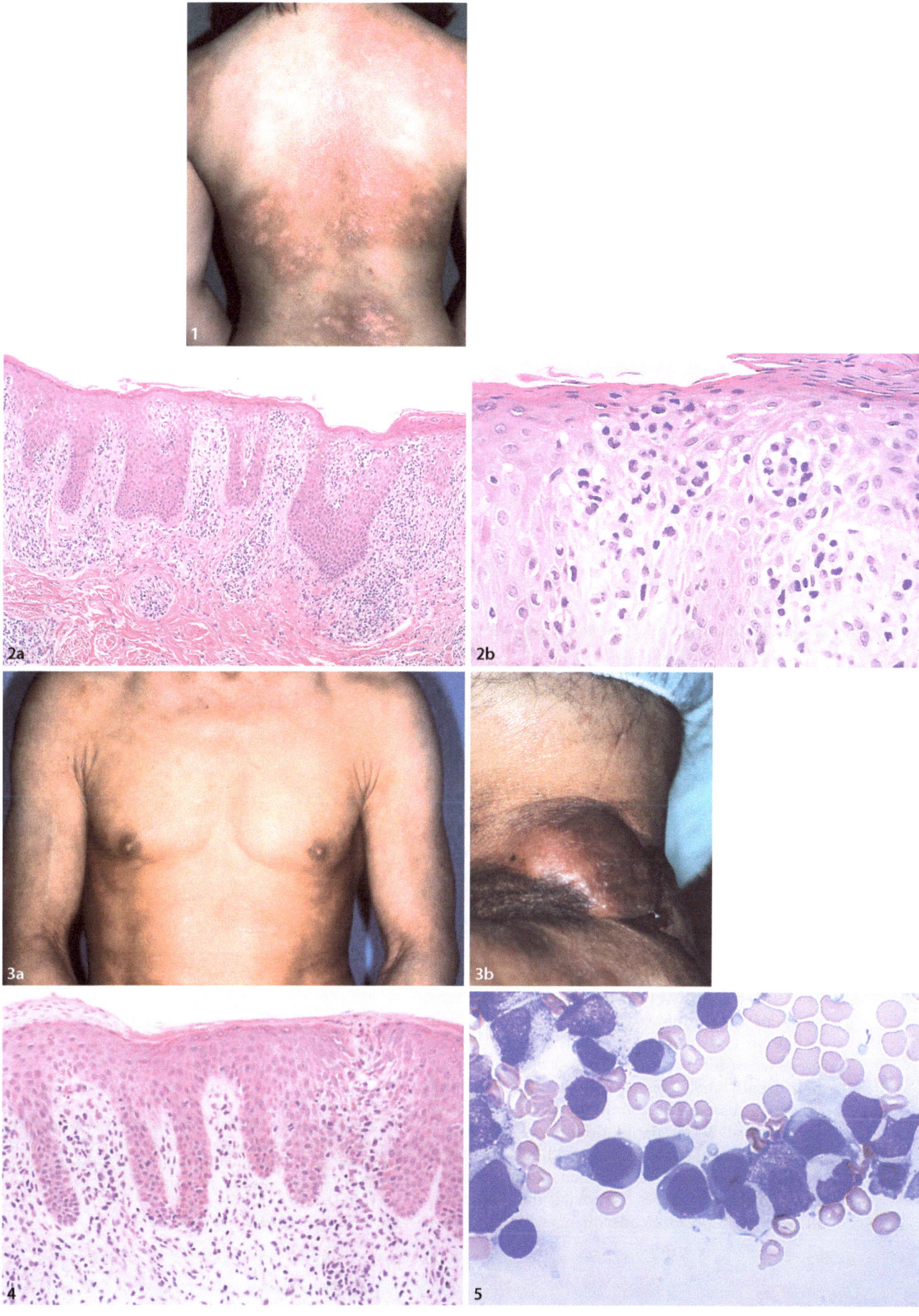

A case of mycosis fungoides with polyarthritis showing clonal identity in skin and synovial tissue

Y. SANDBERG, A. W. LANGERAK and F. HEULE

Age: 57 years **Sex:** M

Clinical features: This patient was known with a 12-year history of psoriasiform skin lesions, which had been diagnosed histopathologically as eczema. At presentation the lesions had further progressed and clinical examination demonstrated enlarged inguinal lymph nodes. A new skin biopsy specimen demonstrated a dense infiltrate of atypical CD4$^+$ T-cells with epidermotropism. Isolated atypical T-cells appeared to have a typical cerebriform nucleus by electron microscopy. Histopathological examination of a lymph node showed features of dermathopathic lymphadenopathy. Patient was treated with class II corticosteroid creams in combination with UVB therapy, showing a temporarily positive effect on the skin lesions.

Diagnosis: Mycosis fungoides (MF), stage II.

Follow-up: Five years after presentation a symmetric erosive polyarthritis of wrists, small hand joints and feet developed and he was diagnosed with rheumatoid factor-negative rheumatoid arthritis (RA). A synovial biopsy specimen demonstrated a large dense infiltrate of small mature T-lymphocytes (CD45RO$^+$). Patient was treated with NSAID's, DMARD's and methotrexate. His condition exacerbated and he developed widespread tumor-stage disease. T-cell receptor (TCR) gene rearrangement analysis was performed on DNA extracted from both skin and synovial tissue and demonstrated clonal identity. Patient refused more aggressive multiagent chemotherapy and later he became progressively systemically ill with B-symptoms. He died 11 years after presentation.

Comment: This case illustrates the prolonged clinical course of MF through many stages. Five years after the diagnosis of MF was made, the patient developed a chronic erosive polyarthritis, which could be classified as RA. Polyarthritis in the presence of MF is rare and may involve different pathogenic mechanisms which have recently been discussed. The finding of an identical monoclonal T-cell population in skin and inflamed synovial tissue illustrates "homing" of circulating lymphoma cells, which might enhance inflammation. Besides, synovial dissemination of MF has important consequences for therapy.

Fig. 1: Large indurated plaque with ulcerations and underlying lymphadenopathy of the right upper leg and groin.

Fig. 2: Skin biopsy demonstrating an infiltrate of atypical lymphocytes with alignment along the basal layer of the epidermis and epidermotropism consistent with the diagnosis MF. HE, microscopic magnification 100×.

Fig. 3: Electronmicroscopic image of an atypical lymphocyte with cerebriform nucleus (N), isolated from a skin lesion.

Fig. 4: Hand showing signs of arthritis deformans.

Fig. 5: Roentgenogram of the hands, demonstrating radiar deviation of the carpus and ulnar deviation of the fingers, periarticular osteoporosis, joint space narrowing and joint erosions. The arrows point at joint erosions.

Fig. 6: Histology of synovium. Localization of an infiltrate composed of predominantly small round nucleated mature lymphocytes (arrows) with a slight propensity for alignment along vessels (V). HE, microscopic magnification 400×.

Fig. 7: Southern blot analysis of *TCRB* genes of skin and synovial tissue. Upon hybridization with the TCRBJ2 probe in an *Eco*RI digest, a clear clonal non-germline band is observed in the skin sample; the same band in synovial DNA indicates clonal identity of the T-cell population in both tissues. G: germline band.

References

van Doorn R, Van Haselen CW, van Voorst Vader PC, Geerts ML, Heule F, de Rie M, Steijlen PM, Dekker SK, van Vloten WA, Willemze R (2000) Mycosis fungoides: disease evolution and prognosis of 309 Dutch patients. Arch Dermatol 136:504–510

Sandberg Y, El Abdouni M, Lam KH, Langerak AW, Lugtenburg PJ, Dolhain RJ, Heule F (2004) Clonal identity between skin and synovial tissue in a case of mycosis fungoides with polyarthritis. J Am Acad Dermatol 51:111–117 *

* Case description reprinted from J Am Acad Dermatol 2004;51:111–117; Sandberg Y, El Abdouni M, Lam KH, Langerak AW, Lugtenburg PJ, Dolhain RJ, Heule F; Clonal identity between skin and synovial tissue in a case of mycosis fungoides with polyarthritis, with permission from the American Academy of Dermatology, Inc.

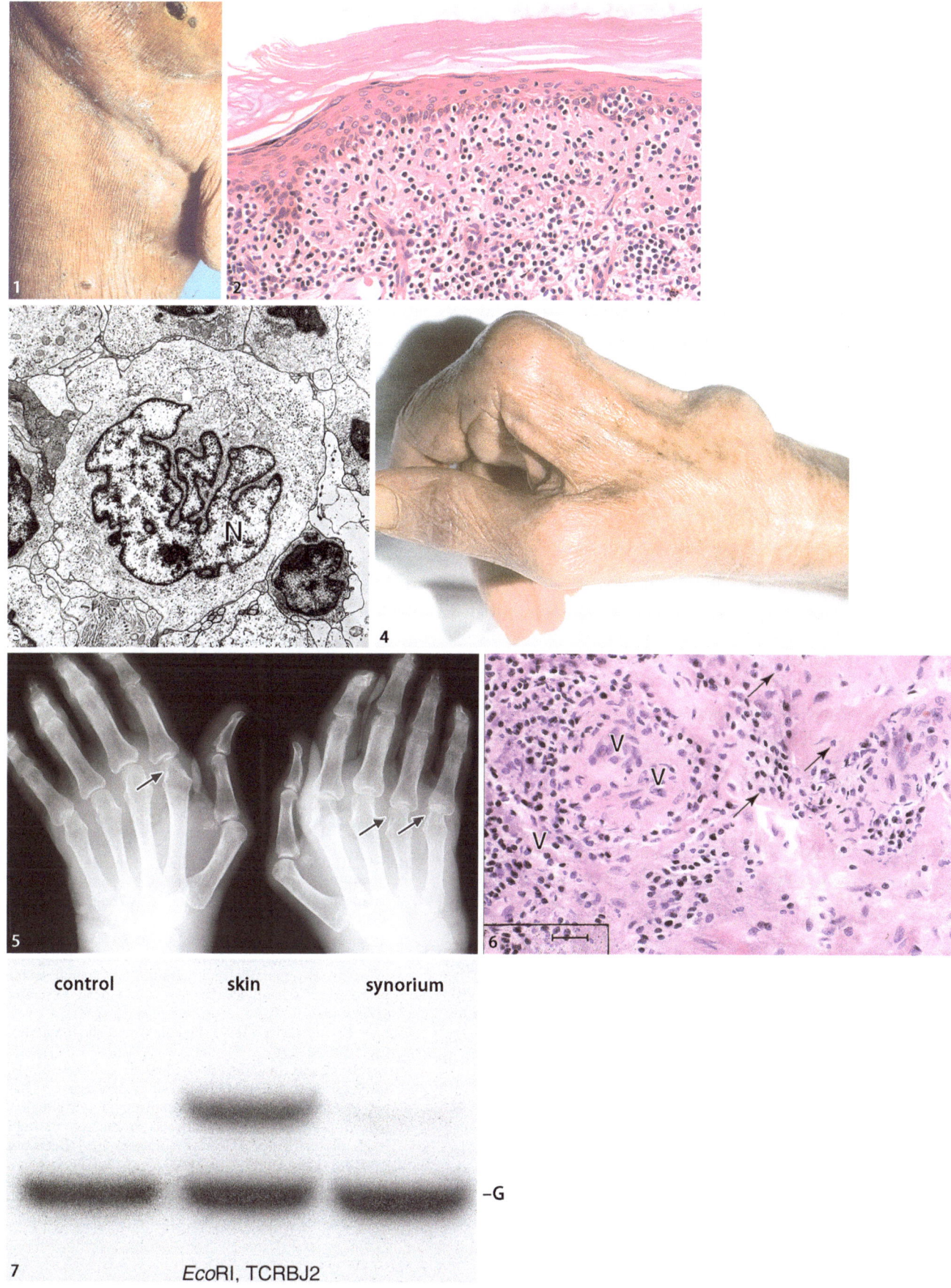

Vesicular mycosis fungoides

M. H. Vermeer, M. W. Bekkenk, P. M. Jansen, C. J. M. Meijer and R. Willemze

Age: 62 years   **Sex:** M

Clinical features: The patient presented with a generalized eruption of sharply demarcated, erythematous plaques. Within these plaques and on erythematous skin small vesicles with yellow content were observed. One year before presentation the skin lesions had started in the presternal region and had then spread to the trunk and extremities. Tzanck smear, potassium hydroxide preparation, viral cultures and bacterial cultures of the pustules were negative. There was no lymphadenopathy. Peripheral blood counts were without abnormal findings.

Diagnosis: Vesicular mycosis fungoides.

Follow-up: Photochemotherapy with 8-methoxypsoralen in combination with clobetasol-propionaat ointment once a day resulted in a partial remission.

Two years after diagnosis involvement of inguinal, axillary and mediastinal lymph nodes developed and CHOP-chemotherapy was initiated. After two cycli of chemotherapy the patient developed a generalized herpes zoster infection. Despite intensive treatment he died 10 days later.

Comment: Mycosis fungoides presenting with vesicular lesions is unusual and provides a diagnostic challenge. Patients with vesiclular mycosis fungoides lesions limited to the hands and feet have been described as mycosis fungoides palmaris et plantaris. The clinical features including small vesicles and pustules with yellowish scale crust, sometimes accompanied by nail dystrophy, can be indistinguishable from those of palmoplantar pustulosis or dyshidrotic eczema. Mycosis fungoides patients with a more generalized pustular eruption on the trunk and extremities have also been described. Histologically, there are intra-epidermal spaces filled with a variable proportions of atypical cells, neutrophils and eosinophils. Production of IL-8 by the neoplastic cells has been suggested to play a role in the development of vesicular/pustular lesions in mycosis fungoides. Depending on the clinical context differential diagnosis includes: palmoplantar pustulosis, Sneddon-Wilkinson disease, pustular psoriasis, bacterial and viral infections, and immunobullous disorders.

In mycosis fungoides patients presenting with larger, blistering and erosive plaques and tumors the differential diagnosis should include aggressive CD8-positive, epidermotropic CTCL. To complicate matters, bacterial or viral superinfections in mycosis fungoides lesions may lead to development of pustules and/or vesicles. Especially patients with folliculotropic mycosis fungoides frequently develop bacterial super-infections. Moreover, all patients on local or systemic immunosuppressive therapy have an increased risk on herpes infections as was dramatically illustrated in this patient. In addition, a pustular folliculitis caused by Demodex mites has been reported in a patient with mycosis fungoides during total-skin electron beam therapy.

- **Fig. 1:** Generalized eruption of sharply demarcated, erythematous plaques with small vesicles and crustae.
- **Fig. 2:** Numerous small vesicles within an erythematous plaque.
- **Fig. 3 and Fig. 4:** Infiltration of the epidermis by atypical lymphocytes with convoluted nuclei and blasts.
- **Fig. 5:** Staining for CD3 demonstrates extensive infiltration of the epidermis by neoplastic cells.

References

Moreno JC, Ortega M, Conejo-Mir JS, Sanchez-Pedreno P (1990) Palmoplantar pustulosis as a manifestation of cutaneous T cell lymphoma (mycosis fungoides) J Am Acad Dermatol 23:758–759

Toritsugi M, Satoh T, Higuchi T, Yokozeki H, Nishioka K (2004) A vesiculopustular variant of mycosis fungoides palmaris et plantaris masquerading as palmoplantar pustulosis with nail involvement. J Am Acad Dermatol 51:139–141

Camisa C, Aulisio A (1994) Pustular mycosis fungoides. Cutis 54:202–204

Poszepczynska E, Martinvalet D, Bouloc A, Echchakir H, Wechsler J, Becherel PA, Boumsell L, Bensussan A, Bagot M (2001) Erythrodermic cutaneous T-cell lymphoma with disseminated pustulosis. Production of high levels of interleukin-8 by tumour cells. Br J Dermatol 144:1073–1079

Nakagawa T, Sasaki M, Fujita K, Nishimoto M, Takaiwa T (1996) Demodex folliculitis on the trunk of a patient with mycosis fungoides. Clin Exp Dermatol 21:148–150

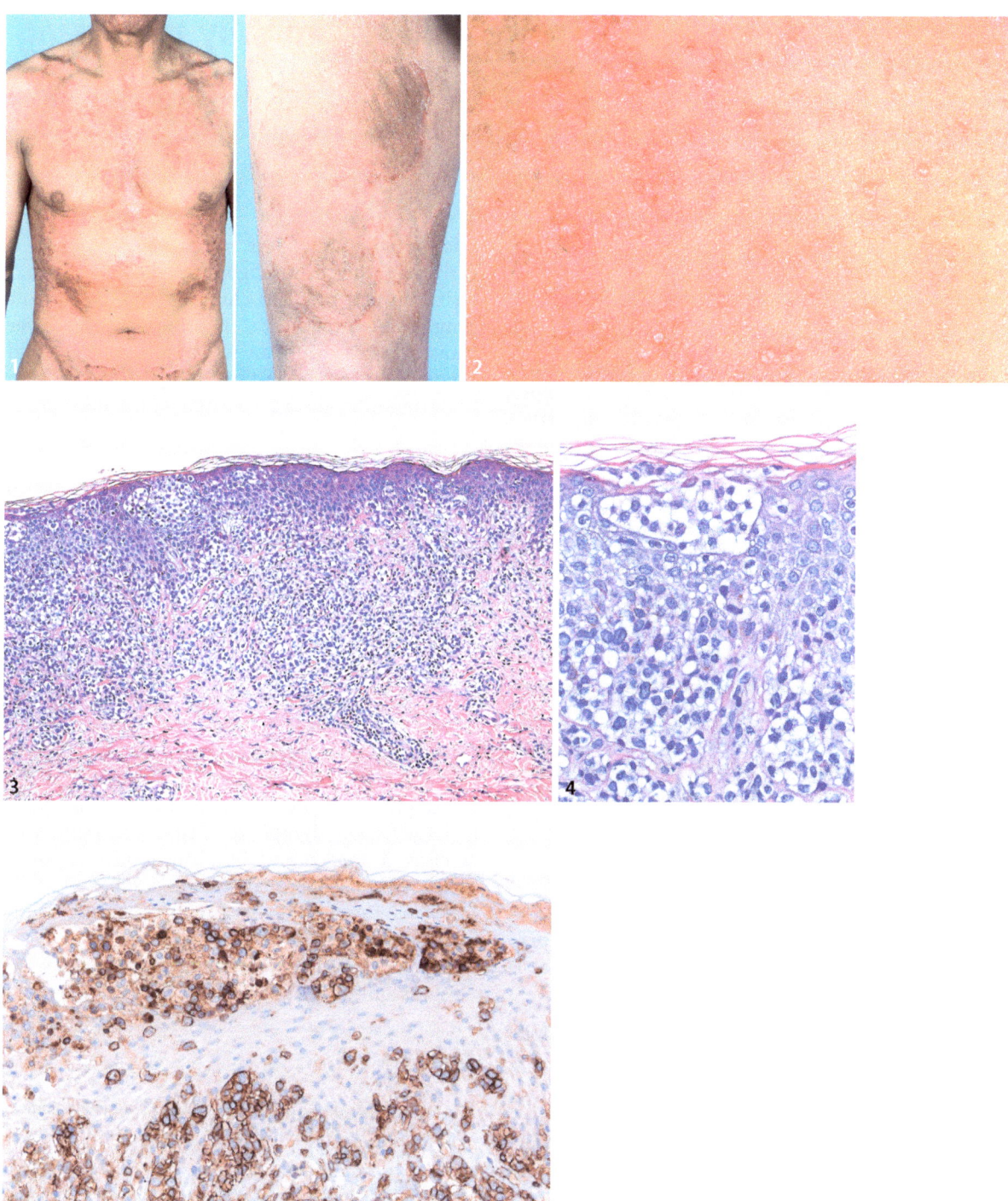

Unusual case of mycosis fungoides clinically mimicking a dermatophytosis subsequently evolving in aggressive CD30– cutaneous lymphoma

L. Citarella and S. Chimenti

Age: 35 years   **Sex:** F

Clinical features: A 35 years old woman referred to our Department because of the presence since several months of some slightly pruritic lesions localized at lower limbs and unresponsive to systemic and topic antifungal therapy. Laboratory investigation for mycotic infection was negative and haematochemical findings were within normal limits. A skin biopsy specimen revealed typical epidermotropic cutaneous lymphoma early stage and gene-rearrangement detected monoclonality of T-cell receptor. Monochromatic excimer laser (MEL 308 nm) treatment was performed with initially partial response. During the treatment several large tumours developed *de novo* on the scalp. A skin biopsy specimen of one of these tumours showed histological and immunophenotypical features of a medium-large sized pleomorphic T-cell lymphoma. The patient was firstly unsuccessfully treated with CHOP-regimen chemotherapy. Subsequently vinorelbine and gemcitabine were administrated achieving after 8 cycles a complete remission of cutaneous manifestations.

Diagnosis: Mycosis fungoides transient in primary cutaneous pleomorphic medium/large T cell CD30– lymphoma.

Follow-up: Clinical remission obtained is still maintained after 6 months of follow-up.

Comment: Early stage mycosis fungoides was reported to simulate different dermatological disorders, including dermatophytosis. We report this case to stress the importance to be aware of the possibility that in some cases patch lesions apparently benign could be overlooked with a delay in diagnosis and management. Furthermore, this paradigmatic case reminds that, even if early stage mycosis fungoides usually is characterized by an indolent clinical course with slow progression over years, in some cases however transformation into an aggressive entity could occur in a short period of time. The progression into tumour stage is associated with a poor prognosis and a low survival rate.

Fig. 1: Large lesion with annular borders, slightly rilevated and mildly scaling clinically resembling dermatophytosis.

Fig. 2: Histology picture of biopsy from the leg: epidermis shows fibrinoid material and exocytosis of lymphocytic elements. The dermal infiltrate is represented by atypical lymphoid elements with hyperchromatic nuclei. HE, Microscopic magnification 40×.

Fig. 3: Large and multilobated tumours developed *de novo* on the scalp.

Fig. 4: Histology picture of biopsy from the scalp: in the dermal pleomorphic medium-large sized lymphoid cells infiltrate with cleaved nuclei and atypical mitotic figures. HE, Microscopic magnification 200×.

Fig. 5: Immunohistochemistry staining demonstrated a CD3 positive infiltrate.

Fig. 6: Complete remission of cutaneous lesions on the scalp.

References

Kazakov DV, Burg G, Kempf W (2004) Clinicopathological spectrum of mycosis fungoides. J Eur Acad Dermatol Venereol 18:397–415

Willemze R, Kerl H, Sterry W et al. EORTC (1997) Classification for Primary cutaneous Lymphomas: A Proposal from the Cutaneous Lymphoma Study Group of the European Organization for Research and Treatment of Cancer. Blood 90:354–371

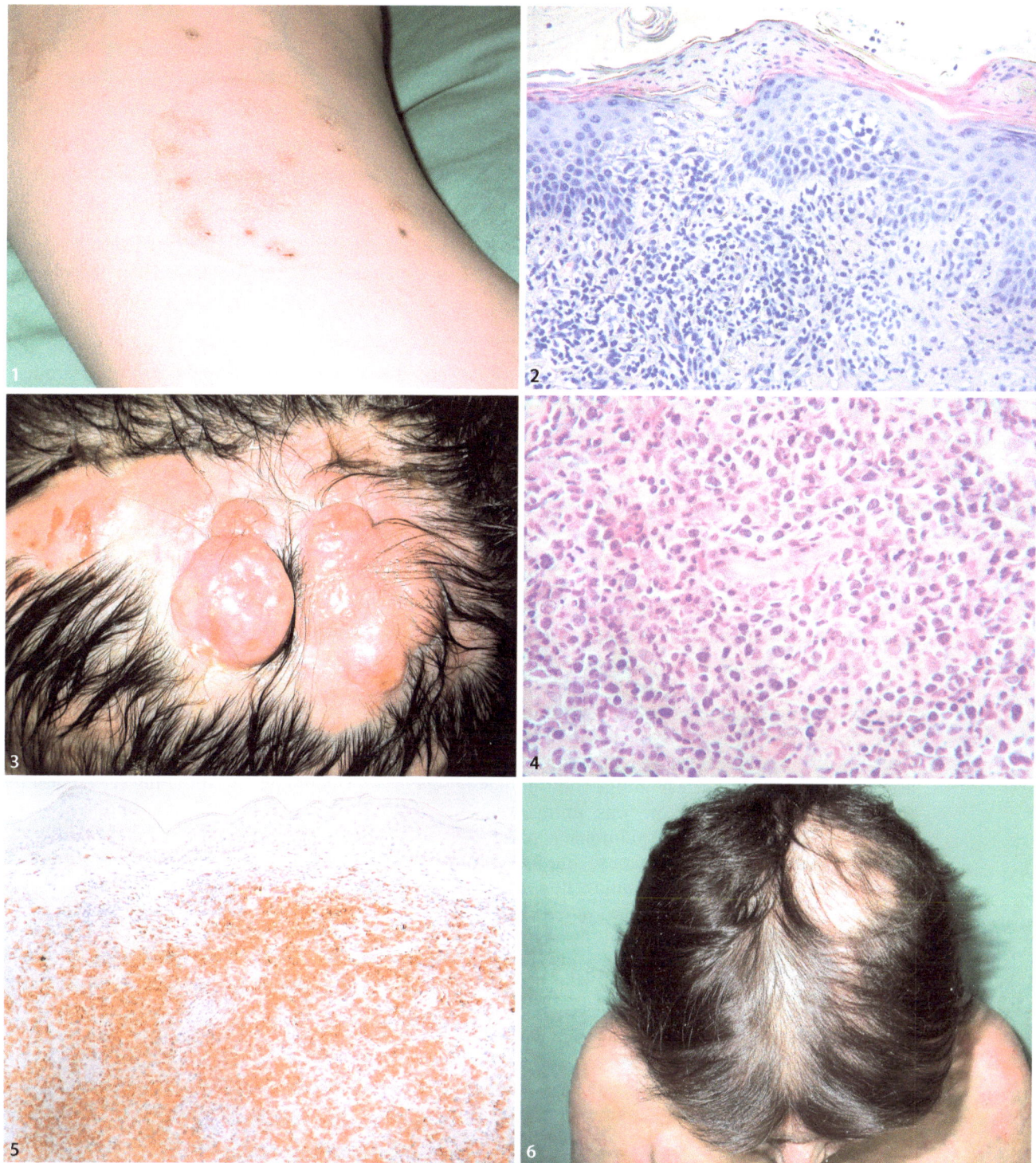

Sclero-atrophic mycosis fungoides with a cytotoxic atypical phenotype

M. G. Bernengo, P. Quaglino and M. Novelli

Age: 58 years   **Sex:** M

Clinical features: Previous diagnosis of follicular Mycosis fungoides (MF) in 1996, treated with long-term P-UVA therapy at another institution. Recent appearance of sclerodermiform lesions, associated to the development of superficial adenopathies, fever and dyspnoea. The patient presented with slightly erythematous scaling patches and papules associated with multiple infiltrated plaques and nodules, located predominantly to the trunk and upper limbs, characterized by a sclerodermic and atrophic appearance, and frequently surrounded by an erythematous ring; superficial adenopathies up to 10 cm in diameter were palpable. The cutaneous biopsy showed an atypical lymphoid CD2+CD3+CD5−CD4−CD8− TIA1+γ/δ+ cell infiltrate. The nodal biopsy showed a complete effacement by large confluent clusters of atypical cells sharing the same atypical phenotype found in the skin. The PCR analysis showed a dominant TCR- gene rearrangement in both skin and node specimens. Laboratory examinations revealed markedly increased LDH values; antinuclear and extractable nuclear antigen antibodies were negative. Bone marrow was uninvolved, whereas CT scan showed a pulmonary parenchymal mass; the percutaneous fine-needle biopsy revealed a chronic granulomatous process and Klebsiella pneumoniae was isolated from the bronchoalveolar fluid.

Diagnosis: γ/δ+ stage IV ($T_3LN4M_0B_0$) MF with sclero-atrophic features.

Follow-up: Systemic polichemotherapy with a standard CHOP regimen was carried out, associated with antibiotics. At the time of writing, the disease is stable after two courses, whereas the lung CT scan shows a complete clearing of the pneumonia infection.

Comment: Cutaneous γ/δ+ lymphoma represent an extremely rare CTCL subtype, not yet included in the WHO/EORTC classification, characterised by a predominant involvement of the extremities with plaques, tumours and panniculitis-like subcutaneous nodules, by a frequent CD4−CD8+ or CD4−CD8− cytotoxic phenotype with T-cell lineage antigen loss, and by a generally aggressive clinical course. In our patient, the medical history suggests and the clinico-pathologic data steer into a MF rather than a peripheral T-cell lymphoma, even if the phenotype at first diagnosis was not available. The interest of our case lies also in the unusual clinical sclero-atrophic features. In fact, even if the possible presence of atrophic and/or sclerodermic features have been described in both large plaque parapsoriasis and the so-called poikiloderma atrophicans vasculare (parapsoriasis variegata), only one case of sclerodermiform MF has been reported as far as we know. Even if these prominent features were not primarily present at the first diagnosis, it is unlikely that they could be related to a cutaneous side effect of the long-term photochemotherapy.

- **Fig. 1:** Disseminated sclero-atrophic plaques associated to erythematous patches and papules on the trunk (a) and back (b). Erythematous scaling patches predominate on the lower limbs (c).
- **Fig. 2:** Histology: A thin linear epidermis with thick sclerotic collagen bundles, associated to a diffuse band-like dermal infiltrate with prominent subcutaneous infiltration and rimming of the fat spaces (a). Single-cell epidermotropism along the basal layer (b).
- **Fig. 3:** Immunohistochemistry: CD3 positive (a) TCR γ/δ positive (b) and CD2 positive (c).
- **Fig. 4:** Flow-cytometry on tissue suspension: CD3+ TCR γ/δ+ cells account for about 20% of the lymphoid infiltrate.

References

Toro JR, Liewehr DJ, Pabby N et al. (2003) Gamma-delta T-cell phenotype is associated with significantly decreased survival in cutaneous T-cell lymphoma. Blood 101:3407–3412

Kazakov DV, Burg G, Kempf W (2004) Clinicopathological spectrum of mycosis fungoides. J Eur Acad Dermatol Venereol 18:397–415

Gueguen MH (1971) Mycosis fungoides. A form of pleuro-pulmonary origin with cutaneous sclerodermiform manifestations. Treatment by application of nitrogen mustard. Bull Soc Fr Dermatol Syphiligr 78:617–618

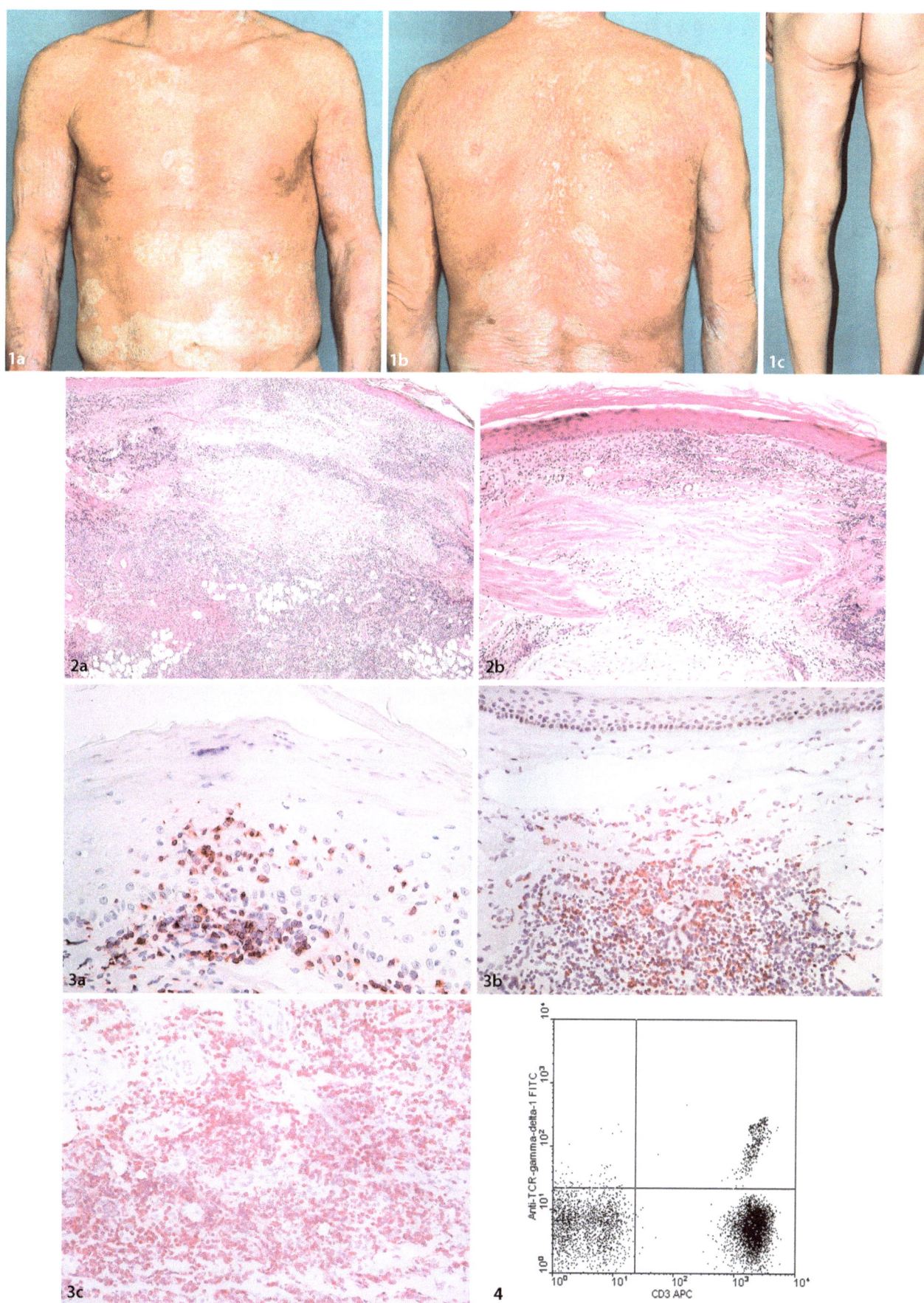

CD56+ early mycosis fungoides

L. CERRONI and H. KERL

Age: 59 years   **Sex:** F

Clinical features: Erythematous patches on the trunk for the last 6 years.

Diagnosis: Early mycosis fungoides with cytotoxic phenotype (γ/δ+, TIA-1+, CD56+).

Follow-up: Complete response to PUVA treatment.

Comment: Early lesions of mycosis fungoides usually show a characteristic CD3+/ CD4+/ CD8– phenotype typical of T-helper lymphocytes. In later stages phenotypic aberrations may occur, including among others development of a cytotoxic phenotype of neoplastic cells (TIA-1+ and/or granzyme-B+). In a very small subset of patients, an unusual phenotype of neoplastic cells is present from the very onset of the disease. The most common phenotypic variant of early mycosis fungoides is characterized by predominance of CD8+ T-cytotoxic lymphocytes. Rarely, a γ/δ +/CD56+ phenotype may be observed in early manifestations of the disease, too. These phenotypic variants usually are characterized by marked epidermotropism and may be the cause of differential diagnostic problems with so-called CD8+ epidermotropic aggressive cutaneous T-cell lymphoma (CTCL) and with cutaneous γ/δ T-cell lymphomas, respectively. These last two entities represent aggressive variants of the CTCLs and bear a poor prognosis. Differential diagnosis is achieved mainly on clinicopathologic correlation: early mycosis fungoides with cytotoxic phenotype reveals the typical patches of the disease, whereas the aggressive CTCLs mentioned above show ulcerated plaques and tumors at onset. Recognition and proper classification of cases of early mycosis fungoides with cytotoxic phenotype is crucial in order to avoid unnecessary aggressive treatment for these patients.

Fig. 1: Erythematous patches of early mycosis fungoides on the trunk.

Fig. 2: Superficial infiltrate with prominent epidermotropism of lymphocytes that are slightly larger than those in the dermis.

Fig. 3: Immunophenotypic features of the epidermotropic lymphocytes: negativity for βF1 (a), positivity for TIA-1 (b) and positivity for CD56 (c).

References

Cerroni L, Gatter K, Kerl H (2004) An illustrated guide to skin lymphoma. 2nd edition. Malden, Oxford, Carlton, Blackwell Publishing

Massone C, Chott A, Metze D et al. (2004) Subcutaneous, blastic natural killer (NK), NK/T-cell, and other cytotoxic lymphomas of the skin. A morphologic, immunophenotypic, and molecular study of 50 patients. Am J Surg Pathol 28:719–735

Tosca AD, Varelzidis AG, Economidou J, Stratigos JD et al. (1986) Mycosis fungoides: evaluation of immunohistochemical criteria for the early diagnosis of the disease and differentiation between stages. J Am Acad Dermatol 15:237–245

Vermeer MH, Geelen FAMJ, Kummer JA et al. (1999) Expression of cytotoxic proteins by neoplastic T cells in mycosis fungoides increases with progression from plaque stage to tumor stage disease. Am J Pathol 154:1203–1210

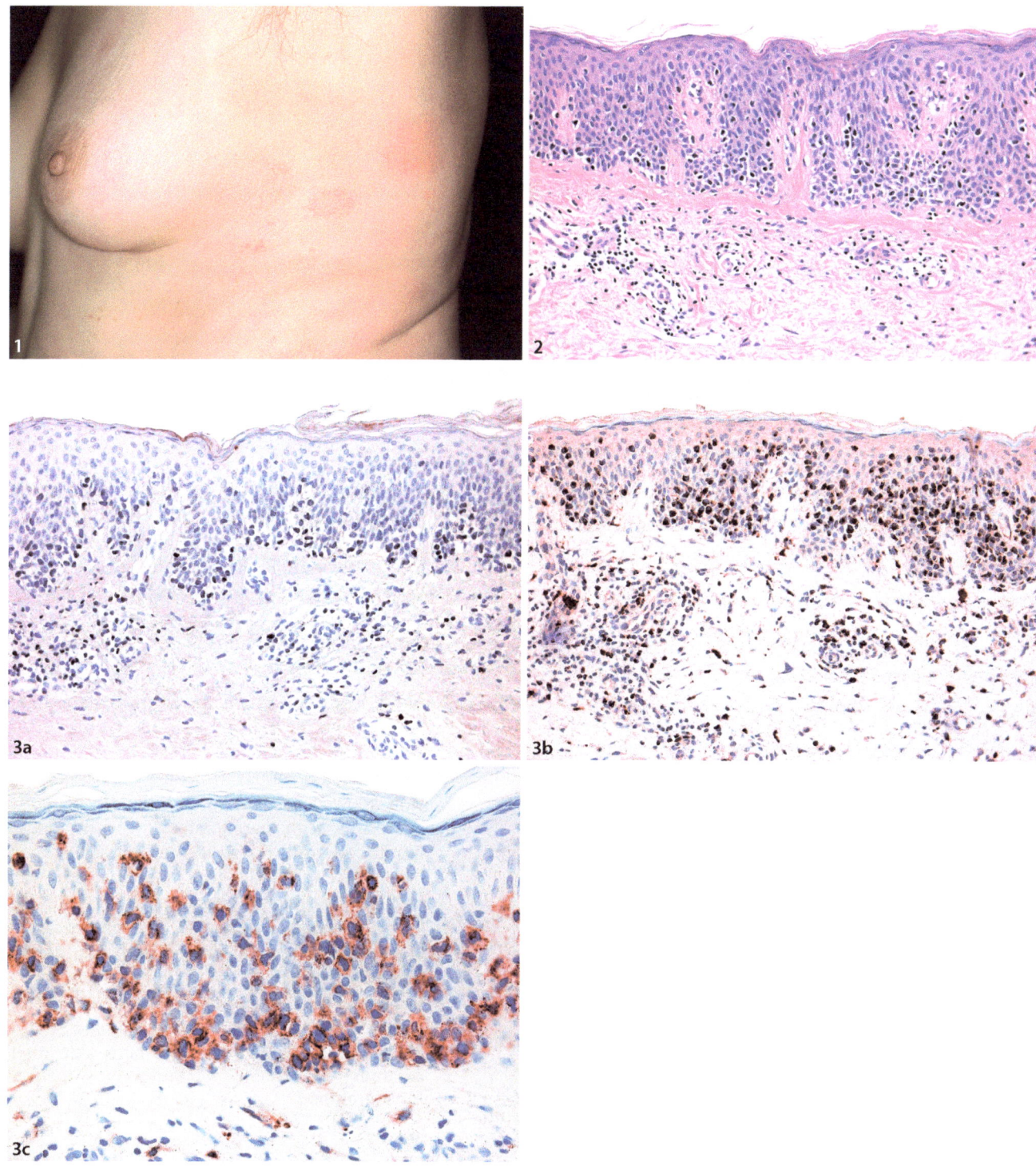

Sézary syndrome with t(2;5) translocation, as developed after prolonged cyclosporine therapy for actinic reticuloid

A. RANKI, L. KARENKO and L. JESKANEN

Age: 62 years   **Sex:** M

Clinical features: The patient had developed UVB sensitivity at the age of 60. Based on clinical lesions on the head and neck and in histopathology, actinic reticuloid was diagnosed. To control the clinical symptoms, oral cyclosporine therapy was started since photoprotection and local therapy had proven unsuccessful. The patient received cyclosporine, with a good clinical response, for one and a half year. At this stage, gyrated skin lesions started to develop on his scalp and neck. Simultaneously, leukocytosis and eosinophilia were observed in peripheral blood: leukocytes 26.5×10^9/l, eosinophils 22% in differential count. Up to 50–60% of peripheral blood lymphocytes had Sézary cell morphology in repeated samples. In peripheral blood lymphocytes, a clonal proliferation was detected based on T-cell receptor rearrangement analysis, and a chromosomal clone with t(2;5) was detected (Karenko et al., unpublished). In a lymph node biopsy, atypical hyperplasia but no clear molecular clones were observed.

Diagnosis: Sézary syndrome (CD3+, CD20–, CD30–).

Follow-up: Cyclosporine therapy was terminated and chlorambucil+prednisone therapy initiated. The latter continued for up to 6 months (with tapering doses of each drug) and a near complete clinical response was achieved. Computed tomography did not show spreading of the lymphoma outside the skin. A relapse occurred after the cessation of the therapy. A RXR-selective retinoid, bexaroten (Targretin) was then started since no phototherapy was possible due to confirmed UVA and UVB sensitivity. The dose was adjusted to 200 mg/m^2 according to serum triglycerin levels (with concomitant atorvastatine 80 mg/d and insulin for diabetes mellitus), and the treatment was maintained for 11 months with partial clinical response. Local electron beam irradiation was given to the remaining CTCL plaques on upper back and shoulder skin. Later, interferon-a (IFN) therapy (starting dose 9 MU×3/week) was combined to bexarotene therapy for another 5 months, and continued alone up to 9 months until an almost complete clinical response was achieved and 20–30% morphological Sézary cells in peripheral blood. No enlarged lymph nodes were found.

Comment: Actinic reticuloid may present in an erythrodermic form, difficult to distinguish from Sezary syndrome. In this patient, however, a clear monoclonal lymphocyte clone could be demonstrated with several methods and the majority of the skin-infiltrating lymphocytes were CD30–. The malignancy was preceded by one and a half years of cyclosporine therapy, and according to current CTCL therapy guidelines, cyclosporine and drugs alike are contraindicated for CTCL therapy.

- **Fig. 1:** The head and neck skin of the patient after 1,5 yrs of therapy with cyclosporine for actinic reticuloid.
- **Fig. 2:** A skin biopsy from a gyrated skin lesion showed acanthotic and slightly oedemic epidermis with parakeratosis (a) and dense lymhocytic infiltration in the dermis (b).
- **Fig. 3:** A few Pautrier-like microabscesses can be found in the epidermis.
- **Fig. 4:** Dermal infiltration is composed of atypical lymphocytes mixed with histiocytes and eosinophils.
- **Fig. 5:** Atypical lymphocytes have convoluted cell membrane and are hyperchromatic.
- **Fig. 6:** The patient's head and neck skin after combined bexarotene and interferon-a therapy for 5 months

References

Bakels V, van Oostveen JW, Preesman AH et al. (1998) Differentiation between actinic reticuloid and cutaneous T-cell lymphoma by T-cell receptor gamma gene rearragement analysis and immonophenotyping. J Clin Pathol 51:154–158

Kadin M, Morris S (1998) The t(2;5) in human lymphomas, Leukemia and Lymphoma 29:249–256

Beylot-Barry M, Groppi A, Vergier B et al. (1998) Characterization of t(2;5) reciprocal transcripts and genomic breakpoints in CD30+ cutaneous lymphoproliferations. Blood 91:4668–4676

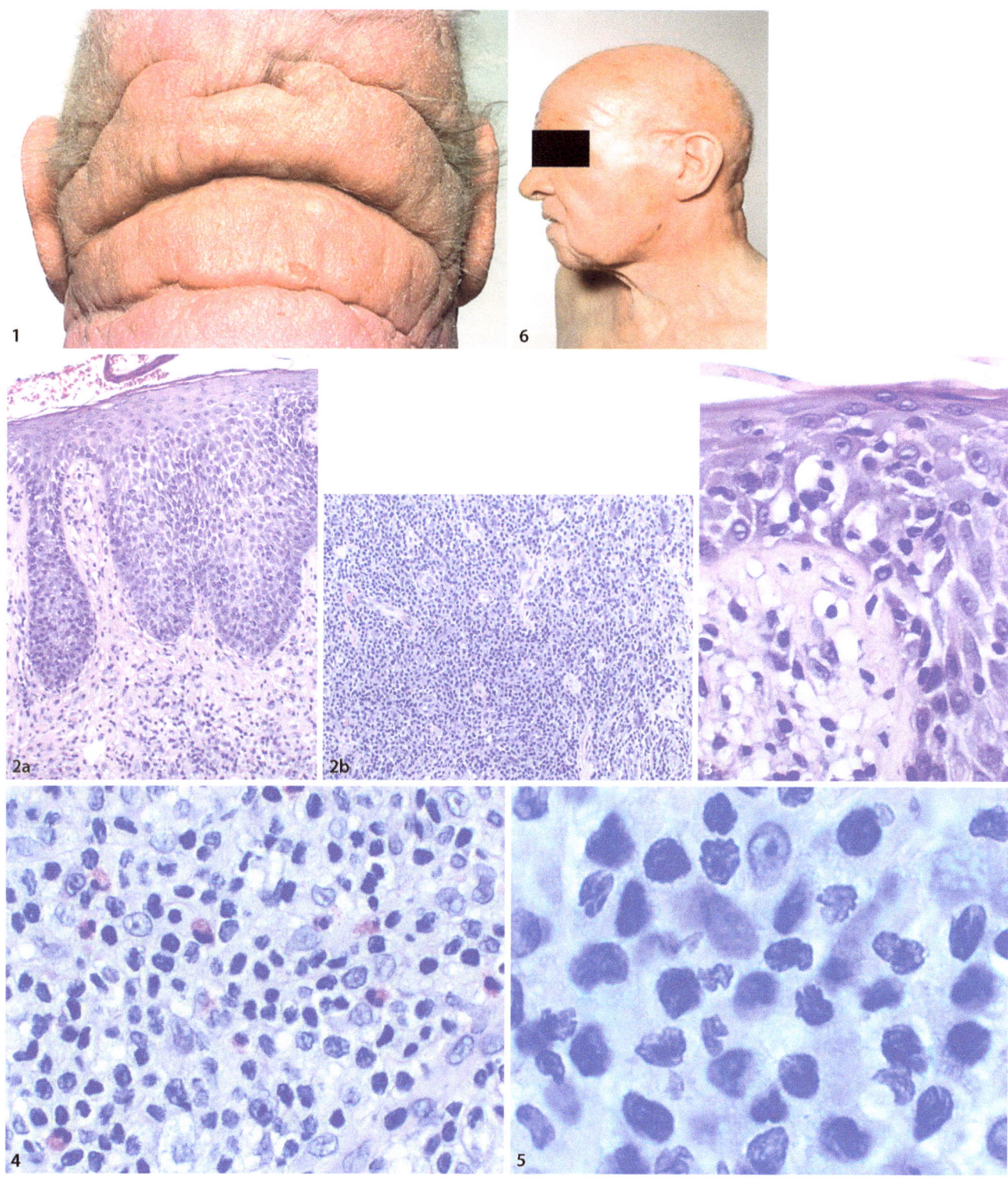

■ CD8+ Lymphomatoid papulosis with simultaneous Type A, Type B, and Type C lesions

J. J. ABBOTT, R. H. WEENIG and L. E. GIBSON

Age: 63 years **Sex:** F

Clinical features: One-year history of a relapsing and recurring, pruritic to painful papulonecrotic skin lesions involving the trunk and extremities. The lesions begin as erythematous papules that progress to necrotic papules and nodules, last for a few months and resolve with atrophic hyperpigmented scars. No lymphadenopathy or hepatosplenomegaly was identified on physical exam or CT scan.

Immunoperoxidase stains: Large, atypical lymphoid cells immunoreactive for CD8 and CD30 and non-immunoreactive for CD4.

TCR gene analysis: T-cell clone identified by PCR analysis of the gamma chain on both of 2 biopsies tested.

Diagnosis: CD8+ Lymphomatoid papulosis.

Comment: Lymphomatoid papulosis (LyP) is a cutaneous CD30+ lymphoproliferative disorder characterized by recurrent papulonecrotic or papulonodular skin eruption with histological features of a malignant lymphoma *"lymphomatoid"* and an excellent prognosis (el Azhary et al). The immunophenotype of the atypical lymphoid cells is usually CD4-positive, CD8-negative, CD30-positive, Cytotoxic marker (TIA-1, granzyme B)-positive. CD4-negative, CD8-positive LyP is very rare (Harvell 2002), and has been suggested to be more common in the pediatric population (Aoki 2003). The simultaneous occurrence of type A and type B LyP is reported to occur in up to 9% of patients (Bekkenk 2000). However, simultaneous occurrence of type A, type B, and type C LyP in the same patient is exceedingly rare.

■ **Fig. 1:** Erythematous and necrotic papules and nodules at various stages of evolution.

■ **Fig. 2:** Skin biopsy of early papular lesions showing superficial and deep dermal "wedge-shaped" infiltrate containing large atypical lymphoid cells (Type A LyP). Microscopic magnification 50×, inset 200× (a). Immunoperoxidase stains of skin biopsy above (2A) showing CD8+/CD30+ infiltrate. Microscopic magnification 100× (b).

■ **Fig. 3:** Second skin biopsy showing dense superficial dermal lymphoid infiltrate with extensive epidermotropism (Type B LyP). Microscopic magnification 50×, inset 100× (a). Immunoperoxidase stains of skin biopsy above (3A) showing CD8+ infiltrate with scattered CD30+ cells. Microscopic magnification 100× (b).

■ **Fig. 4:** Third skin biopsy of large necrotic papule (Fig. 1) showing dense diffuse lymphoid infiltrate with dense aggregates of large atypical lymphoid cells (Type C LyP). Microscopic magnification 25× (a). Immunoperoxidase stains of skin biopsy above (4A) showing diffuse CD8+ infiltrate with aggregates of large cells that co-express CD30. Microscopic magnification 50× (b).

References

el-Azhary RA, Gibson LE, Kurtin PJ et al. (1994) Lymphomatoid papulosis: a clinical and histopathologic review of 53 cases with leukocyte immunophenotyping, DNA flow cytometry, and T-cell receptor gene rearrangement studies. J Am Acad Dermatol 30:210–218

Harvell J, Vaseghi M, Natkunam Y et al. (2002) Large atypical cells of lymphomatoid papulosis are CD56-negative: a study of 18 cases. J Cutan Pathol 29:88–92

Aoki E, Aoki M, Kono M, Kawana S (2003) Two cases of lymphomatoid papulosis in children. Pediatr Dermatol 20:146-9

Bekkenk MW, Geelen FA, van Voorst Vader PC et al. (2000) Primary and secondary cutaneous CD30(+) lymphoproliferative disorders: a report from the Dutch Cutaneous Lymphoma Group on the long-term follow-up data of 219 patients and guidelines for diagnosis and treatment. Blood 95:3653-3661

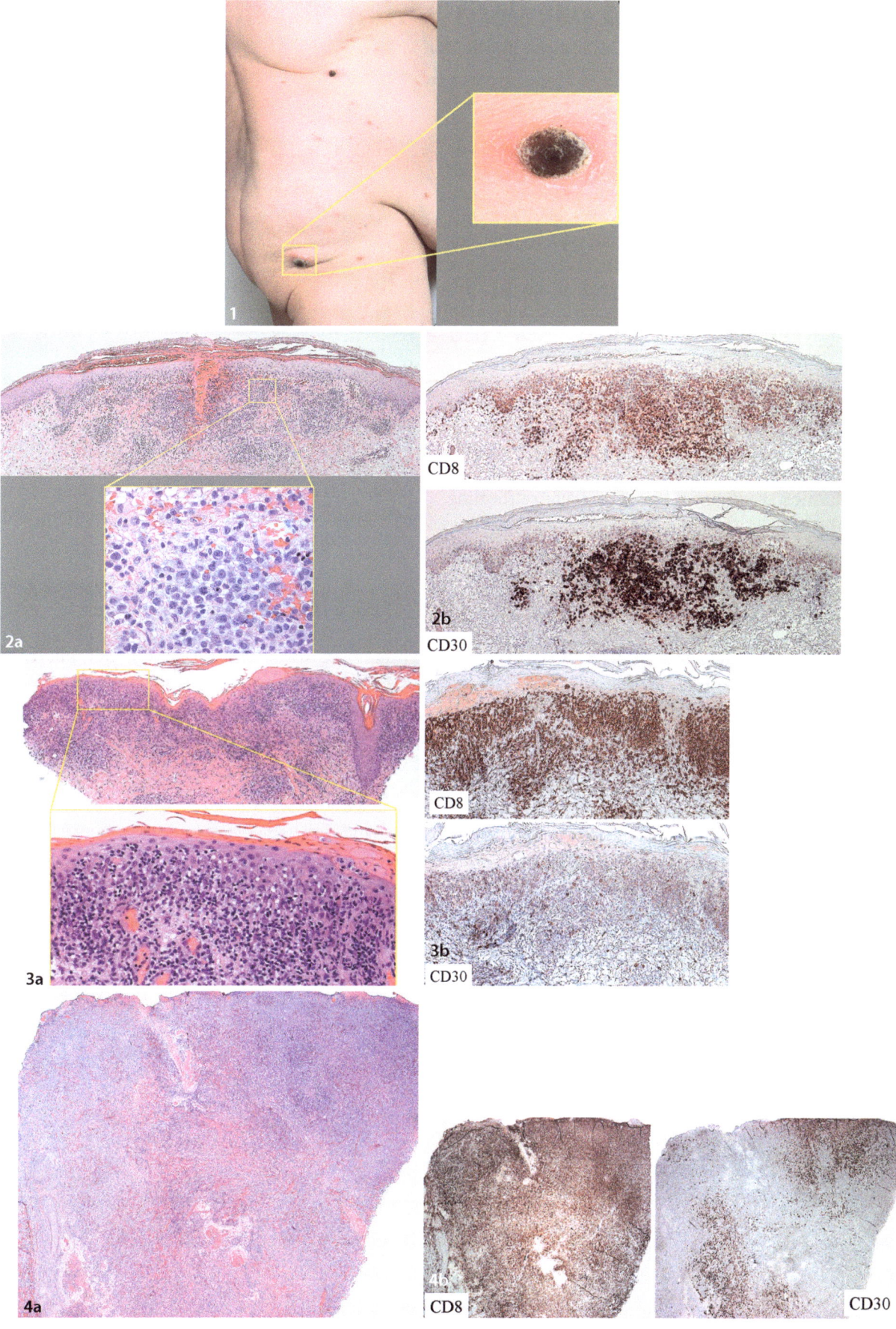

Lymphomatoid papulosis with a NK-cell phenotype

M. W. Bekkenk, C. J. L. M. Meijer and R. Willemze

Age: 47 years   **Sex:** M

Clinical features: A generalized papular skin eruption developed around the age of 27 and had been treated with various topical steroids without effect. The lesions always disappeared spontaneously after 6–8 weeks, but new lesions appeared at other sites simultaneously. Recently a larger tumorous lesion appeared on his leg, but also showed spontaneous resolution. Skin biopsy showed a dense infiltrate with CD3–/CD30+/CD56+ atypical cells. A thoracic and abdominal computed tomographic scan, bone marrow biopsy, blood analysis and an examination by an ear/nose/throat specialist were performed, but these failed to demonstrate extracutaneous involvement. Clinical observation during hospitalization confirmed the recurrent, selfhealing nature of the skin lesions.

Diagnosis: Lymphomatoid papulosis, with a natural killer-cell phenotype.

Follow-up: When treatment with low-dose oral methotrexate (22,5 mg weekly) was instituted, no further lesions developed and the existing lesions slowly resolved. Methotrexate was tapered off and our patient remains free of skin lesions on a maintenance dose of 10 mg weekly.

Comment: Detailed immunophenotypical and genotypical analysis indicated that the atypical cells in this patient were of true NK-cell origin rather than T cells coexpressing CD56. The absence of TCR-gamma chain gene rearrangement cannot be attributed to underrepresentation of too low a number of CD30+/CD56+ atypical cells, as these constituted approximately 50% of the total number of cells in the dermal infiltrate. Clinically the patient showed classical features of LyP, with a history of 20 years of waxing and waning of papulonodular lesions. Whereas staging is usually not indicated in patients with LyP, we decided to stage this particular patient because of the extent and size of the skin lesions, the uncertainty at the first visit whether there was complete clearance of all individual lesions, and in particular the uncommon phenotype of the atypical cells, given that CD56+ non-Hodgkin's lymphomas are usually associated with a poor prognosis. In two recent reviews on CD56+ neoplasms presenting in the skin CD30-expression was a good prognostic factor. Although co-expression of CD56 is rare in CD30+ lymphoproliferations, the prognosis appears not to be different from "normal" CD56-negative cases. In our view these CD56+ cases would, at least a part of them, best be classified as CD30+ lymphoproliferations and treated similarly.

- **Fig. 1:** Multiple papular lesions coalescing to form a large plaque on the abdomen.
- **Fig. 2:** Dense infiltrate of atypical cells (a) expressing CD30 (b), CD56 (c), but not CD3 (d). Original Microscopic magnification 200×.

References

Bekkenk MW, Kluin PM, Jansen PM et al. (2001) Lymphomatoid papulosis with a natural killer-cell phenotype. Br J Dermatol 145:318–322

Bekkenk MW, Jansen PM, Meijer CJ, Willemze R (2004) CD56+ hematological neoplasms presenting in the skin: a retrospective analysis of 23 new cases and 130 cases from the literature. Ann Oncol 15:1097–1108

Gniadecki R, Rossen K, Ralfkier E, Thomsen K, Skovgaard GL, Jonsson V (2004) CD56+ lymphoma with skin involvement: clinicopathologic features and classification. Arch Dermatol 140:427–436

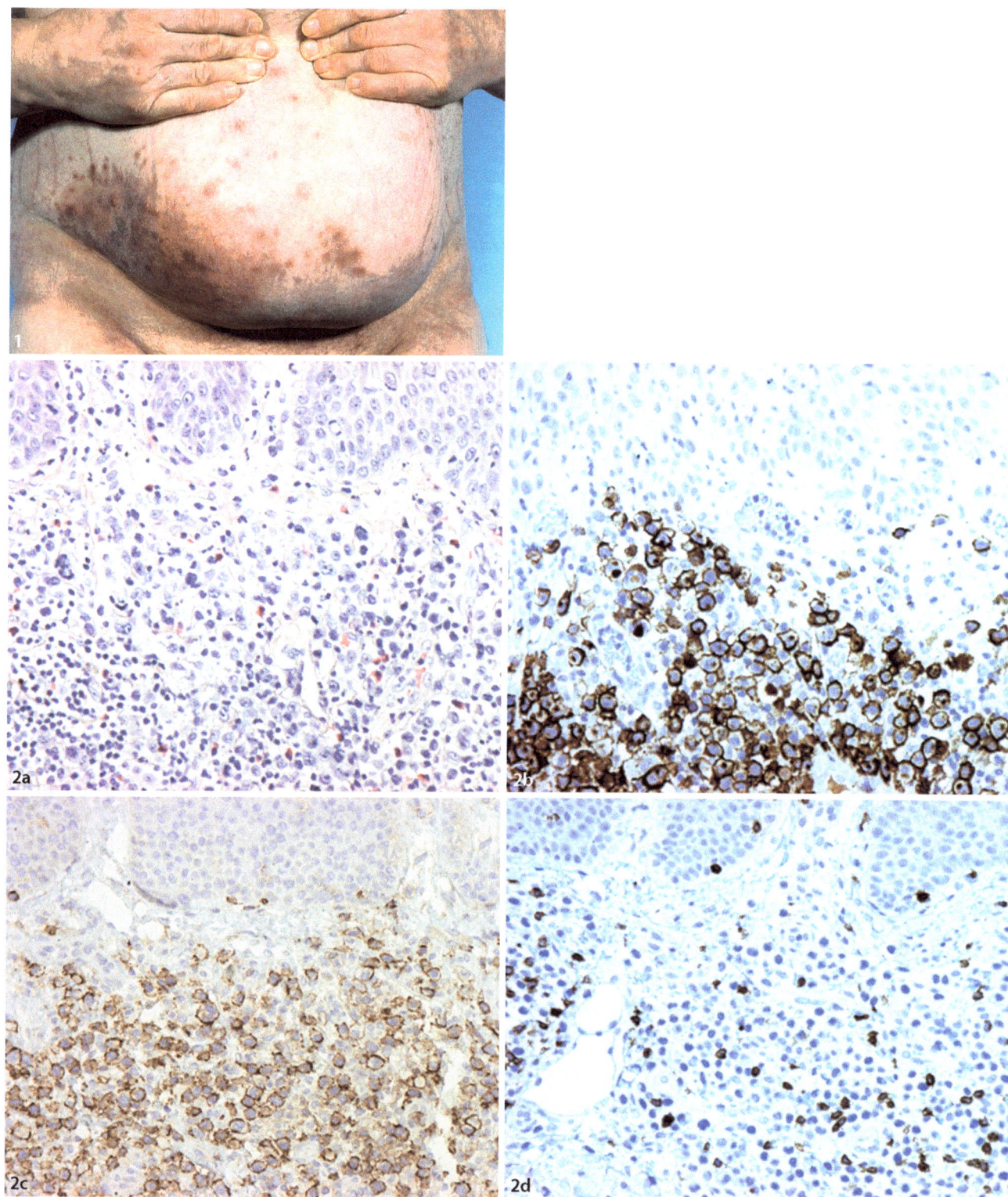

Anaplastic large cell lymphoma associated with acquired ichthyosis

H. Matsuura and S. Morizane

Age: 58 years   **Sex:** M

Clinical features: An ulcerated erythematous nodule on the nose and pigmented ichthyosiform eruption on the trunk had been present for one year. Enlarged lymph nodes were palpable in the submandibular and cervical regions. Organomegaly was not observed. Peripheral blood counts and blood chemistry tests were within normal limits. The majority of tumor cells in the nodular lesion were positive for CD30 and negative for ALK protein. T cell receptor β gene rearrangement was detected by Southern blotting analysis. The ichthyosiform lesion showed no infiltration of atypical cells.

Diagnosis: CD30-positive anaplastic large cell lymphoma (ALCL) associated with acquired ichthyosis.

Follow-up: The nodule on the nose had cleared after three courses of the multiagent chemotherapy with cyclophosphamide, doxorubicin, vincristine, and prednisolone (CHOP), followed by electron beam therapy (total 40 Gy). Three years later, subcutaneous nodules occurred on the buttock associated with inguinal lymph node swelling. Additional three courses of CHOP therapy achieved complete remission. The ichthyosiform eruption did not respond to the chemotherapy.

Comment: Acquired ichthyosis occurs in association with malignant lymphoproliferative disorders, including Hodgkin's disease and other lymphoproliferative disorders such as ALCL (Banerjee et al. 1991) (Kato et al. 2000) and lymphomatoid papulosis (Yokote et al. 1994). It is intriguing to note that acquired ichthyosis is associated with lymphoid malignancies characterized by the presence of CD30-positive neoplastic cells. An ichthyosiform variant of mycosis fungoides should be distinguished from acquired ichthyosis, because of the presence of epidermotropic infiltration of atypical cells in the ichthyosiform lesions. A pathogenesis of acquired ichthyosis in lymphoproliferative disorders remains unclear, although it has been considered that impaired vitamin A metabolism or epidermal lipogensis may be involved. In contrast to cases with Hodgkin's disease, the ichthyosiform eruption was not improved after treatments in our case. Acquired ichthyosis may be an important sign of underlying malignant lymphoproliferative disorders, including ALCL.

Fig. 1: An erythematous nodule with ulcer on the dorsum of the nose.

Fig. 2: Ichthyosiform eruption on the trunk.

Fig. 3: Histpathologic appearance of the nodule on the nose: the infiltrate consists of large lymphoid cells with prominent nuclear polymorphism. HE, microscopic magnification 200×.

Fig. 4: The neoplastic cells are strongly positive for CD30 in the membrane and cytoplasm. Microscopic magnification 400×.

Fig. 5: Ichthyosiform lesion shows compact orthokeratosis with a few granular cell layer and a sparse infiltrate of mononuclear cells without atypical cells. HE, microscopic magnification 200×.

Fig. 6: T-cell receptor β gene rearrangement by Southern blot hybridization. Rearranged bands are detected after restriction enzyme digestion with Bam HI (lane 1), Eco RI (lane 2), or Hind III (lane 3). Red arrows indicate rearranged bands, a) normal control; b) patient.

References

Banerjee SS, Heald J and Harris M (1991) Twelve cases of Ki-1 positive anaplastic large cell lymphoma of skin. J Clin Pathology 44:119–125

Kato N, Yasukawa K, Kimura K et al. (2000) Anaplastic large-cell lymphoma associated with acquired ichthyosis. J Am Acad Dermatol 42:914–920

Yokote R, Iwatsuki K, Hashizume H et al. (1994) Lymphomatoid papulosis associated with acquired ichthyosis. J Am Acad Dermatol 30:889–892

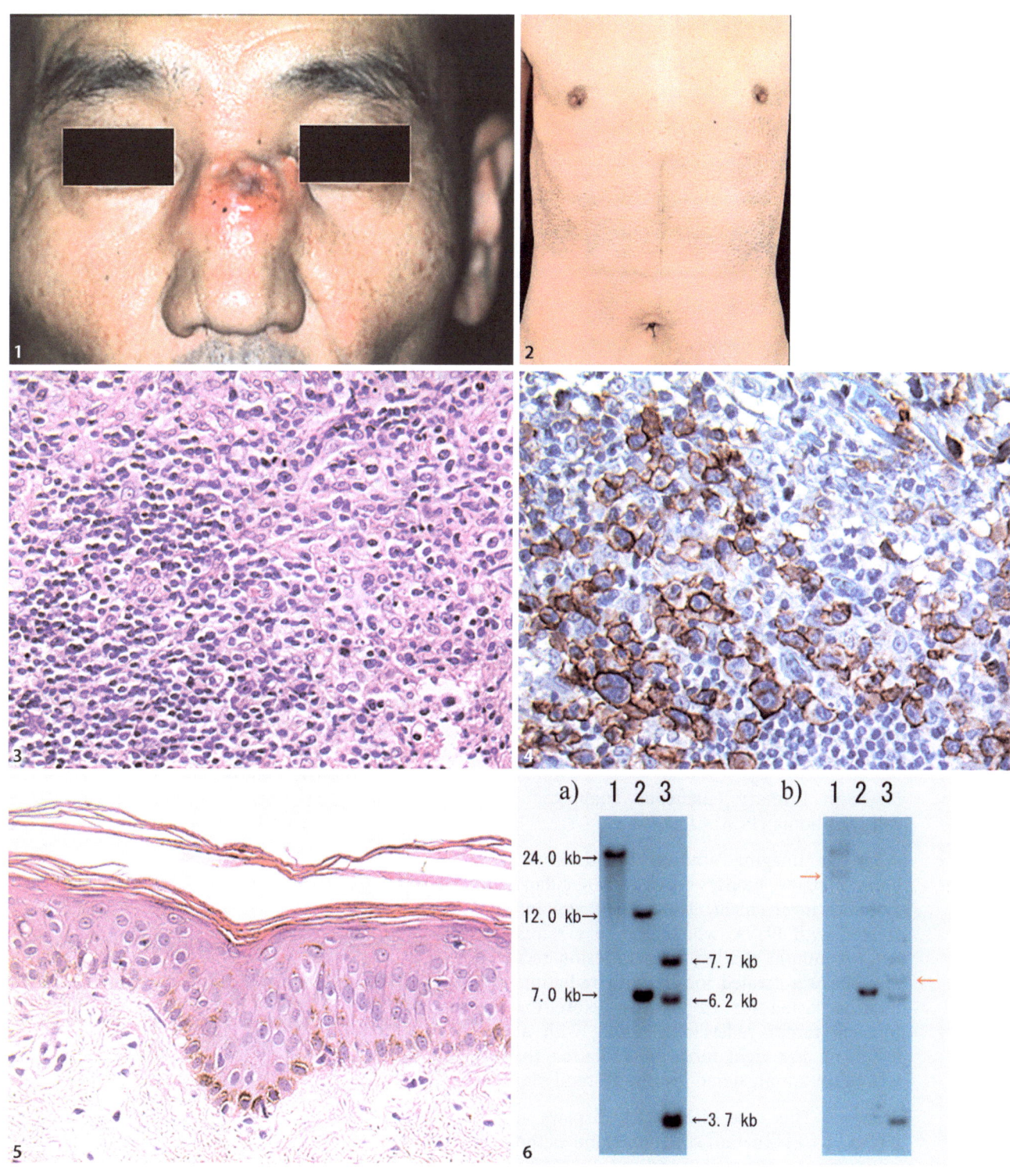

Anaplastic large cell T-cell lymphoma

A. SEKULIC, R.H. WEENIG, I. AHMED and M.R. PITTELKOW

Age: 73 years   **Sex:** F

Clinical features: Patient presented with a 5-year history of largely asymptomatic, annular, migrating and self-resolving patches and plaques involving her extremities. Initial treatment with topical and systemic corticosteroids at home provided temporary relief. Three skin biopsies were obtained at the referring institution and interpreted as mycosis fungoides. Treatment with topical nitrogen mustard was initiated twice and both times discontinued within a few days due to a severe local reaction. On presentation, annular to serpiginous, erythematous plaques with fine scaling were observed on her arms, thighs and buttock. A large erythematous tumor with superficial erosion and serous drainage was present on her left forearm. Two skin biopsies were obtained and both demonstrated a dense dermal lymphoid infiltrate with epidermotropism and clusters of large, anaplastic lymphoid cells. Greater than 75% of the anaplastic large cells were positive for CD30 antigen. In addition, review of the initial biopsies from the referral institution also showed greater than 75% of the large atypical lymphoid cells were CD30-positive.

Diagnosis: Primary cutaneous anaplastic large cell lymphoma (PCALCL).

Follow-up: Imaging studies, blood work and bone marrow biopsy showed no evidence of systemic involvement. The patient was initially treated with PUVA, which lead to a remission. After 4 months the left forearm lesion recurred and she was treated locally with radiation. Remission lasted for 18 months before the left forearm tumor redeveloped along with a new lesion on her right forearm. Radiation therapy was again administered leading to remission.

Comment: This case of PCALCL displays an interesting combination of clinical and pathological features. Although localised PCALCL portends good prognosis, multi-site disease has been linked to a more aggressive behavior and is often treated by systemic chemotherapy (Howard L Liu et al. 2003). Our patient illustrates a case of multifocal PCALCL with a benign clinical course in absence of systemic therapy. Histologic features marked by significant epidermotropism are suggestive of transformed mycosis fungoides (Vergier B et al. 2000). However, persistent CD30 expression with benign clinical behavior favours a diagnosis of a clinically indolent form of multifocal PCALCL.

- **Fig. 1:** Patches, plaques and tumors on patients arms (**a**, **b**) and legs (**c**).
- **Fig. 2:** Skin biopsy of a plaque on the left forearm demonstrated diffuse, atypical dermal lymphocytic infiltrate with epidermal collections of lymphocytes (**a**, **b**, **c**). The large atypical cells expressed CD30 marker (**d**).
- **Fig. 3:** Southern blot analysis for TCR gene rearrangements. Cells were isolated from the forearm lesion and sorted using magnetic beads coupled to CD30 and CD4 antibodies. Molecular genetic studies for TCR gene rearrangements on sorted cell populations demonstrated an identical clonal rearrangement in both CD4 and CD30 positive cells. This confirmed that CD30 positive cells were truly neoplastic and not merely a reactive infiltrate.

References

Howard L Liu, Hoppe RT, Kohler S et al. (2003) CD30+ cutaneous lymphoproliferative disorders: The Stanford experience in lymphomatoid papulosis and primary cutaneous anaplastic large cell lymphoma. J Am Acad Dermatol 49:1049–1058

Vergier B, de Muret A, Beylot-Barry M et al. (2000) Transformation of mycosis fungoides: clinicopathological and prognostic features of 45 cases. French Study Group of Cutaneious Lymphomas. Blood 95(7):2212–2218

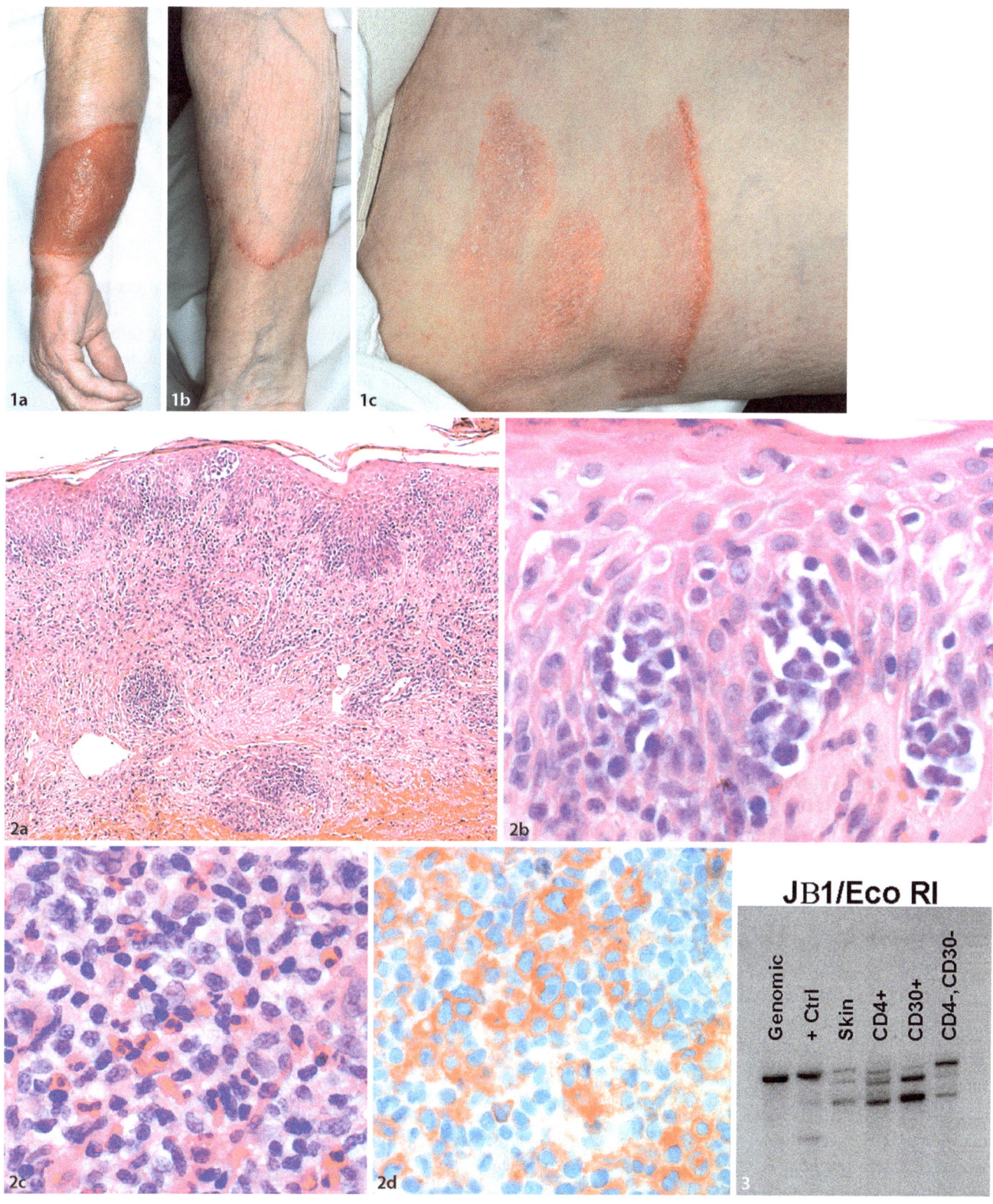

Primary cutaneous histiocyte and neutrophil rich CD30+/CD56+ anaplastic large cell lymphoma of the scalp with prominent angio- and neuroinvasion

L. Boudova, D. V. Kazakov, P. Mukenšnabl, V. Kuntscher and M. Michal

Age: 57 years   **Sex:** F

Clinical features: The patient consulted a neurologist because of headache. During the next three months a tumour spread rapidly over the whole right half of her neurocranium, showing vast skin ulcerations, purulent secretion, massive soft tissue destruction, and incipient bone involvement.

Diagnosis: Primary cutaneous histiocyte and neutrophil rich CD30+/CD56+ anaplastic large cell lymphoma (ALCL).

Follow-up: The immunocompetent patient was administered six cycles of chemotherapy (CHOP), and proceeded to high-dose chemotherapy with autologous peripheral blood stem cell transplantation as a remission consolidation. She has remained in complete remission for more than six years.

Comment: Primary cutaneous neutrophil-rich ALCL is very rare. Occurring predominantly on the head, it is characterized histologically by a large number of neutrophils which may obscure the anaplastic or pleomorphic tumour cells. Initially thought to be associated with HIV infection, it has also been found in immunocompetent patients. The dramatic presentation with a rapid growth, purulent discharge ("pyogenic lymphoma"), widespread tissue destruction, but an excellent prognosis seems to be typical.

The presented case carries a remarkable combination of clinicopathological features. Clinically, the tumour infiltration was very extensive and deep. Morphologically, this tumour is not only rich in neutrophils, but histiocytes prevail in the background. Angioinvasion and nerve infiltration are striking. The neoplastic cells coexpress CD30 and CD56, a rare feature representing a dilemma for a precise classification. On immunohistochemistry, the majority of neoplastic cells are also positive for CD7, CD45RO, CD8, granzyme B, TIA-1, and perforin, a few tumour elements express also CD5 and CD43, while ALK1 kinase, epithelial membrane antigen, Epstein-Barr virus (EBV; LMP), CD57, CD138, CD20 and CD79a are negative. Using PCR a monoclonal rearrangement of T-cell receptor gene gamma and absence of DNA of EBV were detected.

■ **Fig. 1:** A non-ulcerated part of the scalp shows a vaguely nodular, pale tumour infiltrate in the dermis with remnants of hair follicles (HE).

■ **Fig. 2:** Geographic necroses in deeper parts of the tumour (HE).

■ **Fig. 3:** Few large anaplastic cells, some resembling Reed-Sternberg cells, in a background of plentiful histiocytes, neutrophils, and small lymphocytes (HE).

■ **Fig. 4:** Histiocytes are the prevailing component (CD68).

■ **Fig. 5:** CD30+/CD56+ neoplastic cells scattered individually or in small groups: CD30 (a), CD56 (b).

■ **Fig. 6:** Invasion of blood vessels (a) and nerves (b). The neoplastic cells within the vascular walls and nerves were also CD30+CD56+ (not shown).

References

Boudova L, Kazakov DV, Jindra P, Sima R, Vanecek T, Kuntscher V, Vozobulova V, Bouda J, Michal M (2005) Primary cutaneous histiocyte and neutrophil rich CD30+ and CD56+ anaplastic large cell lymphoma with prominent angioinvasion and nerve involvement in the forehead and scalp of an immunocompetent woman. J Cutan Pathol, accepted for publication Aug 2005

Burg G, Kempf W, Kazakov DV, Dummer R, Frosch PJ, Lange-Ionescu S, Nishikawa T, Kadin ME (2003) Pyogenic lymphoma of the skin: a peculiar variant of primary cutaneous neutrophil-rich CD30+ anaplastic large-cell lymphoma. Clinicopathological study of four cases and review of the literature. Br J Dermatol 148(3):580–586

Jhala DN, Medeiros LJ, Lopez-Terrada D, Jhala NC, Krishnan B, Shahab I (2000) Neutrophil-rich anaplastic large cell lymphoma of T-cell lineage. A report of two cases arising in HIV-positive patients. Am J Clin Pathol 114(3):478–482

Mann KP, Hall B, Kamino H, Borowitz MJ, Ratech H (1995) Neutrophil-rich, Ki-1-positive anaplastic large-cell malignant lymphoma. Am J Surg Pathol 19:407–416

Natkunam Y, Warnke RA, Haghighi B, Su LD, LeBoit PE, Kim YH, Kohler S (2000). Co-expression of CD56 and CD30 in lymphomas with primary presentation in the skin: clinicopathologic, immunohistochemical and molecular analyses of seven cases. J Cutan Pathol 27: 392–399

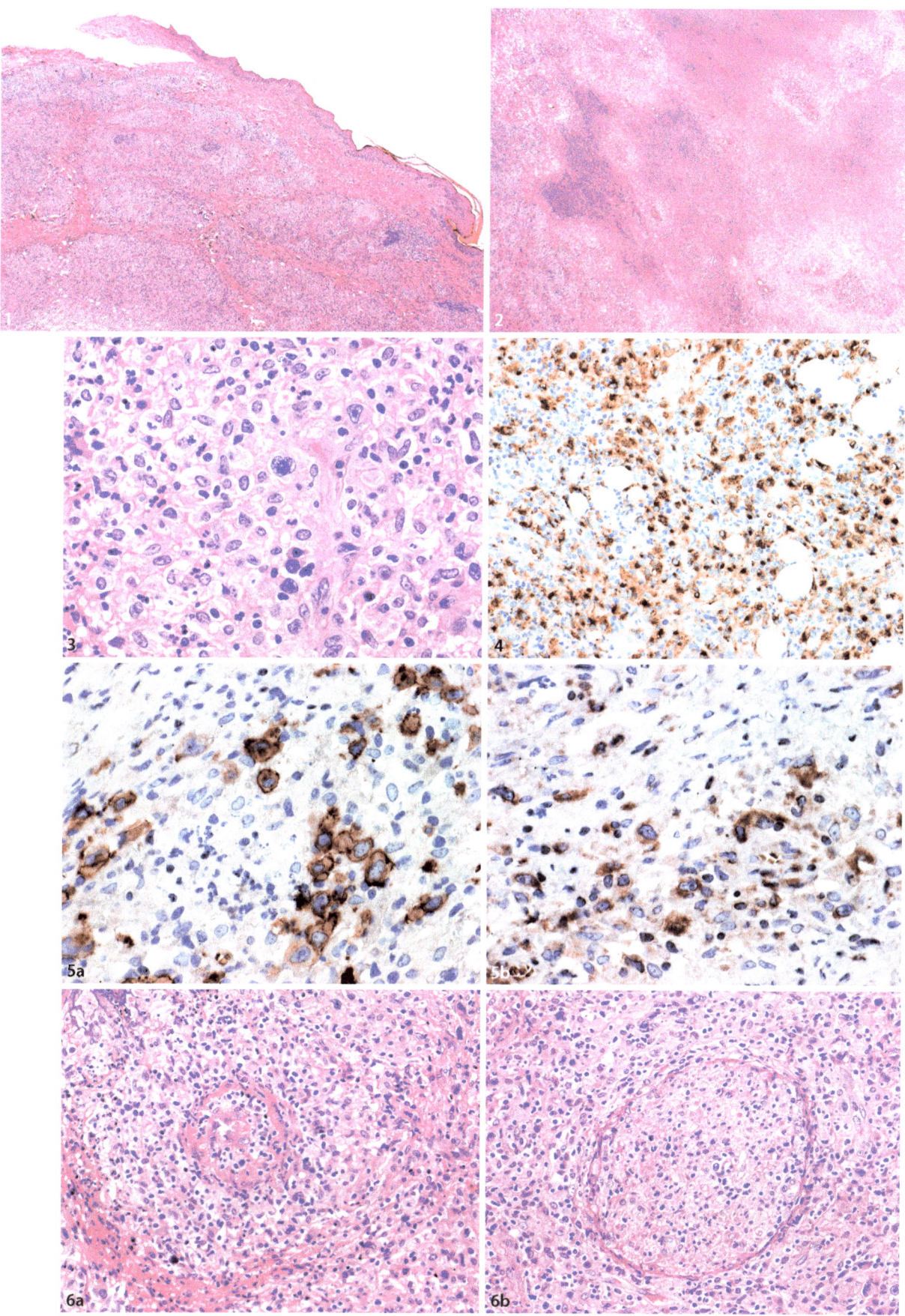

Late relapse of primary cutaneous CD30+ anaplastic large cell lymphoma confirmed by T-cell receptor (TCR) PCR analysis

Y. Sandberg, A. W. Langerak and F. Heule

Age: 47 years   **Sex:** M

Clinical features: A 47 year-old Mediterranean man presented in November 1985 with an ulcerating skin tumor on the left cheek. Histopathological evaluation of a skin biopsy demonstrated a diffuse infiltrate of large polymorphic lymphoid cells, with many mitotic figures and no epidermotropism. Neoplastic cells were strongly positive for CD3 and CD8, and partially CD4+. Complete regression occurred after local radiotherapy (20×2 Gy). Patient did not have any other complaints and dermatological examination did not demonstrate other skin lesions.

Diagnosis: Primary cutaneous anaplastic large cell lymphoma.

Follow up: During follow up patient reported waxing and waning of a few small skin lesions. Spontaneous regression of these lesions occurred in 2–3 months. At the end of 2003, 18 years after initial diagnosis, patient suffered from multiple progressive skin lesions. Dermatological examination demonstrated multiple fleshy nodules and erosive hemorrhagic tumors on the left arm, leg and buttock and partially regressed lesions on the right leg. Multiple skin tumor biopsies all showed localizations of an anaplastic large cell lymphoma. Immunohistochemistry was positive for CD3, CD4, CD8 and CD30 and negative for ALK-1. Molecular clonality analysis demonstrated identical monoclonal *TCRB* gene rearrangements in current skin biopsy specimens and in the initial diagnostic sample, illustrating that the current lesions concern relapses and not secondary or transformed tumors. Immunohistochemical analysis of original biopsy demonstrated large atypical cells, strongly positive for CD30. Staging did not reveal progression to extracutaneous stage of disease. Skin lesions were successfully treated with local radiotherapy (10×2 Gy).

Comment: Although it is known that in patients with primary cutaneous CD30+ anaplastic large cell lymphoma skin lesions may spontaneously regress, a full-blown relapse 18 years after initial diagnosis is extremely rare. This patient illustrates the spectrum of clinical features of CD30+ lymphoproliferative disorders. Although the CD8/CD30 co-expression is rare and is associated with less favorable prognosis, our patient appeared to be in good condition 19 years after initial diagnosis.

- **Fig. 1:** Initial diagnosis. Large ulcerating skin tumor on the left cheek.
- **Fig. 2:** Histology of skin at initial diagnosis. Diffuse infiltrate of large pleomorphic lymphoid cells in the dermis without epidermotropism. HE, microscopic magnification $100\times$; inset, high magnification.
- **Fig. 3:** Neoplastic cells are positive for CD8. Microscopic magnification $200\times$.
- **Fig. 4:** Relapse. Ulcerating tumor with central crust on the left leg, surrounded by multiple fleshy nodules.
- **Fig. 5:** Histology of skin at relapse. Diffuse dermal infiltrate of large atypical lymphoid cells with nuclear pleomorphism. HE, microscopic magnification $100\times$; inset, high magnification.
- **Fig. 6:** The neoplastic cells are strongly positive for CD30. Microscopic magnification $200\times$.
- **Fig. 7:** PCR based GeneScan analysis. Identical monoclonal *TCRB* gene rearrangements were detected in initial diagnostic sample (skin 1985) and recent skin biopsy specimen from tumor (skin I 2003) (a) as well as in skin biopsy from nodule (skin II 2003) Polyclonal *TCRB* gene rearrangements can be identified in control sample (b).

References

Bekkenk MW, Geelen FA, Voorst Vader PC et al. (2000) Primary and secondary cutaneous CD30(+) lymphoproliferative disorders: a report from the Dutch Cutaneous Lymphoma Group on the long-term follow-up data of 219 patients and guidelines for diagnosis and treatment. Blood 95:3653–3661

Berti E, Tomasini D, Vermeer MH et al. (1999) Primary cutaneous CD8-positive epidermotropic cytotoxic T cell lymphomas. A distinct clinicopathological entity with an aggressive clinical behavior. Am J Pathol 155:483–492

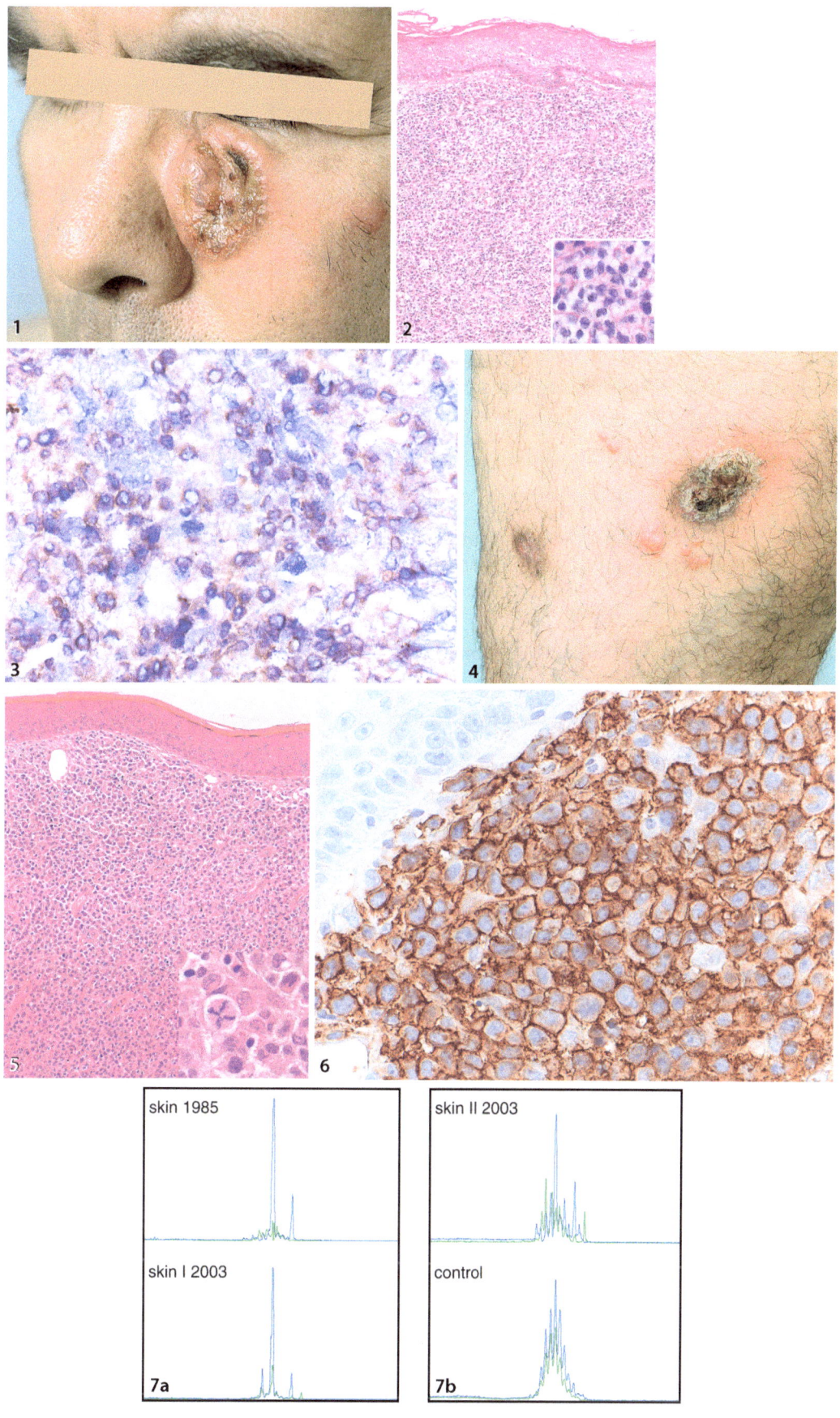

skin 1985

skin II 2003

skin I 2003

control

7a

7b

■ Peripheral CD4+ T-cell lymphoma with cytotoxic phenotype

A. SEKULIC, M. R. PITTELKOW and R. H. WEENIG

Age: 53 years   **Sex:** M

Clinical features: Multiple, asymptomatic subcutaneous nodules have been present on patient's scalp, arms and legs for one year. Some of the lesions have spontaneously regressed in this period and only few have minimal associated ulceration. Staging workup revealed slightly enlarged lymph nodes in supraclavicular, mediastinal, axillary and inguinal areas by CT. PET scan detected only subcutaneous lesions. Clonal T-cell population was detected in subcutaneous nodules (Southern blot) but not in peripheral blood. Bone marrow was normal. All microbial cultures were negative.

Diagnosis: Peripheral T-cell lymphoma, not otherwise specified.

Follow-up: 15 months into the disease, the patient remains stable with slow development of new lesions and spontaneous regression of established nodules.

Comment: This is an unusual case of peripheral T-cell lymphoma that does not fit into existing classification systems (Massone C et al. 2004 and Fink-Puches R et al. 2002.). Pleomorphic, medium to large lymphocytes express markers characteristic of both, helper (CD4) and cytotoxic lymphocytes (TIA-1). Neoplastic cells are negative for CD20, CD30, CD56, Alk-1 and EBV. The absence of staining for CD56 as well as clonal rearrangement of T-cell receptor excludes diagnosis of NK cell lymphoma. This case also lacks characteristic features of panniculitis-like T-cell lymphoma including the karyorrhexis, lipotropism

and panniculitis-like pattern. The unusual clinical course of this lymphoma in form of appearing and spontaneously resolving nodules is interesting in light of the cytotoxic profile of CD4+ lymphoma cells.

■ **Fig. 1:** Subcutaneous nodules on patient's legs (a) and arms (b). Hyperpigmented patches remain in areas of spontaneous resolution (c).

■ **Fig. 2:** Excisional biopsy of a representative subcutaneous nodule demonstrates diffuse lymphohystiocytic infiltrate (a) with large subcutaneous areas of necrosis (b). The infiltrating lymphocytes are medium to large sized and demonstrate cytologic atypia (a).

■ **Fig. 3:** Expression of CD3 marker is detected on the majority of infiltrating cells.

■ **Fig. 4:** Virtually all infiltrating lymphocytes express CD4 antigen.

■ **Fig. 5:** Only scattered CD8 positive cells are noted in the tumor infiltrate.

■ **Fig. 6:** Antibody to TIA-1 stains majority of infiltrating cells suggesting a cytotoxic phenotype.

References

Massone C, Chott A, Metze D et al. (2004) Subcutaneous, blastic natural killer (NK), NK.T-cell, and other cytotoxic lymphomas of the skin. Am J Surg Pathol 28:719–735

Fink-Puches R, Zenahlik P, Back B et al. (2002) Primary cutaneous lymphomas: applicability of current classification schemes (European Organization for Research and Treatment of Cancer, World Health Organisation) based on clinicopathologic features observed in a large group of patients. Blood 99:800–805

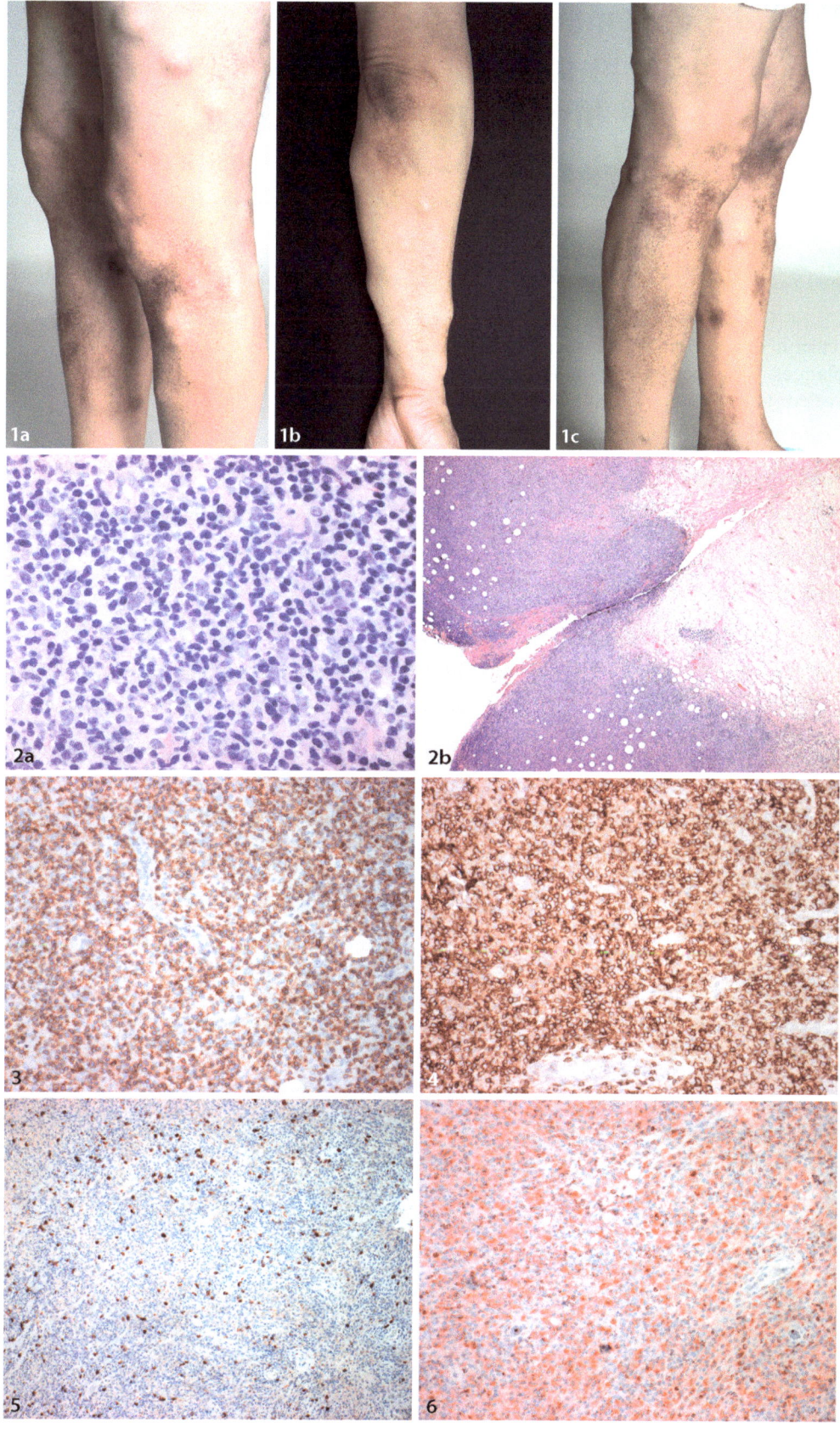

CD8+ disseminated small and medium pleomorphic T-cell lymphoma with blood involvement and secondary hemophagocytic syndrome

M. BAGOT and J. WECHSLER

Age: 92 years **Sex:** M

Clinical features: Onset at 90 years and rapid extension of pruriginous erythematous infiltrated plaques. The peripheral blood cell counts revealed a white blood cell count of 11,500/mL with 12% eosinophils, 6% lymphocytes and 20% atypical lymphocytes with irregular nucleus and cytoplasmic inclusions. Phenotypic analysis of the blood revealed a dominant CD3+CD8+CD45–CD2–CD5–CD7–CD16–CD56– population accounting for 72% of circulating lymphocytes. T-cell-receptor gene analysis showed an identical dominant clone in skin and blood. The blood chemistry test showed increased LDH, beta-2 microglobulin and alkaline phosphatase. No HTLV-1 nor HIV antibodies were detected.

Diagnosis: Disseminated pleomorphic small and medium T-cell lymphoma (CD8+).

Follow-up: He was treated with a combination of local treatment (steroids and chlormethin), chlorambucil (4 mg/day) and low dose prednisone. After 5 months, cutaneous lesions and circulating atypical lymphocytes had disappeared. One month later, occurred a rapidly fatal hemophagocytic syndrome.

Comment: Although our patient had clinical features suggestive of Sézary syndrome, the circulating atypical cells did not have the usual cytological characteristics of Sézary cells, and the dense skin lymphocytic infiltrates were mainly non epidermotropic with numerous interstitial macrophages. Tumor T lymphocytes expressed exclusively CD3 and CD8 and were TIA-1+, Granzyme B–. This patient had a rapidly progressive CD8+ cutaneous lymphoma with blood involvement, and a fatal evolution within less than 6 months.

- **Fig. 1:** Pruriginous erythematous infiltrated plaques.
- **Fig. 2:** Confluent lesions on thorax and abdomen.
- **Fig. 3:** Infiltrated nodules on the arm.
- **Fig. 4:** Dense lymphocytic non epidermotropic infiltrates associated with numerous macrophages (HE, ×100).
- **Fig. 5:** Pleomorphic small and medium T cell lymphoma. HE, microscopic magnification 400×.
- **Fig. 6:** CD68+ macrophagic accessory component. Microscopic magnification 250×.
- **Fig. 7:** CD8+ lymphocytic infiltrates. Microscopic magnification 100×.
- **Fig. 8:** TIA-1+ lymphocytic infiltrates. Microscopic magnification 250×.

References

Agnarsson BA, Vonderheid EC, Kadin ME (1990) Cutaneous T cell lymphoma with suppressor/cytotoxic (CD8) phenotype: identification of rapidly progressive and chronic subtypes. J Am Acad Dermatol 22:569–577

Bekkenk MW, Vermeer MH, Jansen PM et al. (2003) Peripheral T-cell lymphomas unspecified presenting in the skin: analysis of prognostic factors in a group of 82 patients. Blood 102:2213–2219

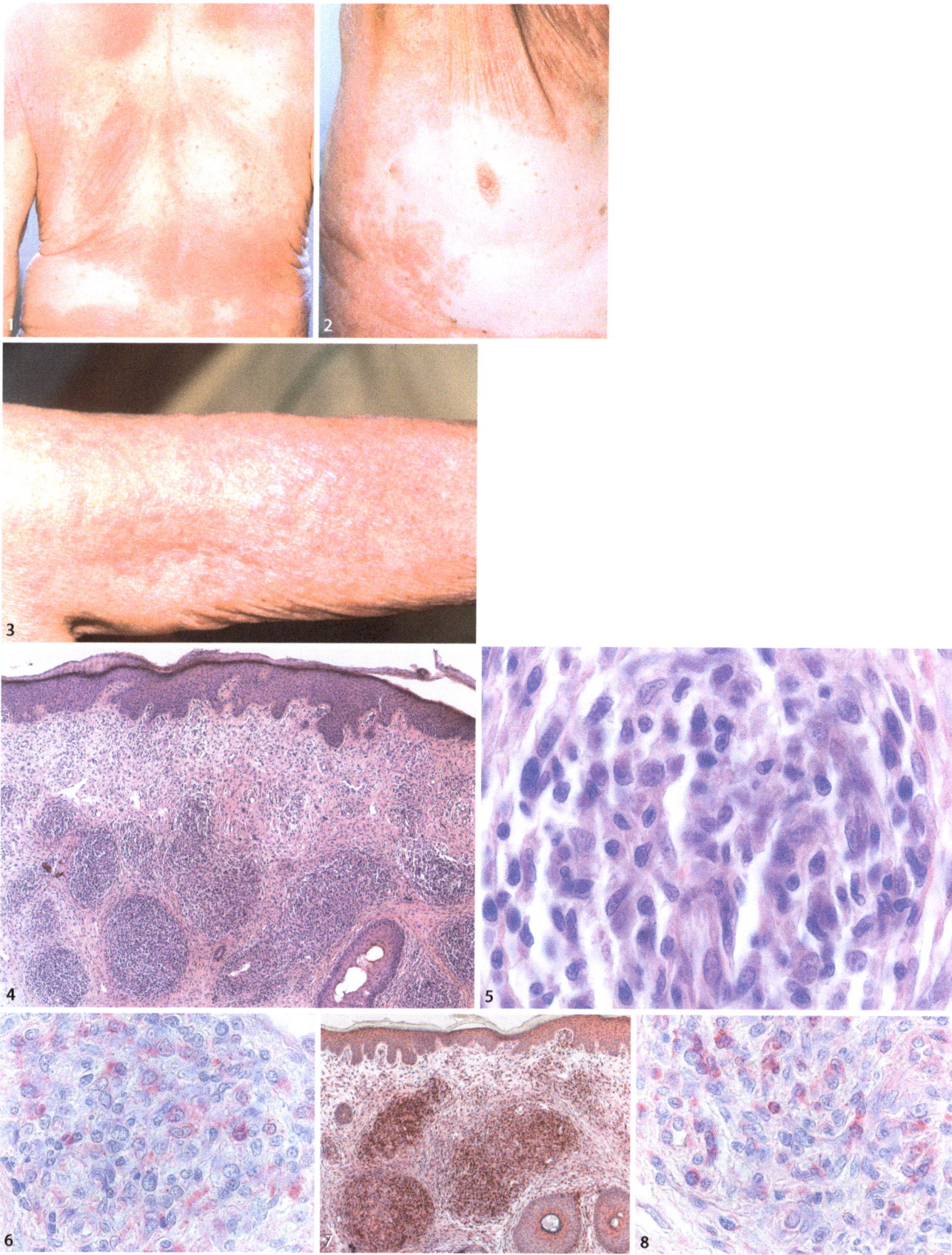

CD8+ cutaneous T-cell lymphoma with an indolent course

B. Laetsch, L. Schärer, G. Burg and R. Dummer

Age: 40 years   **Sex:** M

Clinical features: The patient presented with erythematous plaques on the inner thighs that progressed to nodular infiltrations. A biopsy of this lesions showed small cell T-cell lymphoma, staining for CD 8 showed positivity. Genomic DNA was amplified by polymerase chain reaction. Using primers for $V\gamma 1$–8 and $J\gamma 1/2$ a clonal population was detected.

Diagnosis: CD8+ cutaneous T-cell lymphoma.

Follow-up: The patient was initially successfully treated with PUVA until a relapse after two years. A local therapy with phosphocholin was initiated that lead to a remission within 6 month. This therapy was repeated after another relapse 5 month later and resulted again in a remission. Later the patient was retreated with PUVA. At the moment the disease is stable with local steroid therapy.

Staging procedures by lymphnode and abdominal ultrasound as well as chest x-ray never showed evidence of extracutaneous involvement.

Comment: Cases of CD8+ cutaneous T-cell lymphomas with a benign course have been described before. It is suggested, that CD8+ does not necessarily stand for an unfavourable prognosis, even if the cytotoxicity marker TIA 1 is expressed and suggests cytotoxic T-cell lymphoma. These lymphomas have to be differentiated from other cytotoxic lymphoproliferations and show a nonaggressive clinical behaviour. Therefore they should not be treated aggressively. A highly varying clinical behaviour of CD8+ CTCL was observed by other authors. CD8+ CTCL that were similar to MF, had in general a more rapid disease progression than CD4+ MF. In the case we describe the favourable course doesn't require an aggressive therapy regimen.

Fig. 1: Erythematous to livid, circumscribed plaques on the left thigh medially.

Fig. 2: Biopsy taken at time of initial diagnosis showing a dense infiltrate of small lymphocytes in all dermal layers.

Fig. 3: Exocytosis of small lymphocytes with notched nuclei can be detected at a larger magnification.

Fig. 4: Biopsies taken 5 years later with similar histologic findings.

Fig. 5: Lining up of small atypical lymphcytes in the dermo-epidermal junction zone can be detected.

Fig. 6: Staining for CD 8 showed positivity of the tumor cells.

References

Berti E, Tomasini D, Vermeer MH, Meijer CJ, Alessi E, Willemze R (1999) Primary cutaneous CD8-positive epidermotropic cytotoxic T cell lymphomas. A distinct clinicopathological entity with an aggressive clinical behavior. American Journal of Pathology 155:483–492

Dummer R, Kamarashev J, Kempf W, Haffner AC, Hess-Schmid M, Burg G (2002) Junctional CD8+ cutaneous lymphomas with nonaggressive clinical behavior: a CD8+ variant of mycosis fungoides? Archives of Dermatology 138:199–203

Lu D, Patel KA, Duvic M, Jones D (2002) Clinical and pathological spectrum of CD8-positive cutaneous T-cell lymphomas. [erratum appears in J Cutan Pathol. 2003 Mar; 30(3):222]. Journal of Cutaneous Pathology 29:465–472

Whittam LR, Calonje E, Orchard G, Fraser-Andrews EA, Woolford A, Russell-Jones R (2000) CD8-positive juvenile onset mycosis fungoides: an immunohistochemical and genotypic analysis of six cases. British Journal of Dermatology 143:1199–204

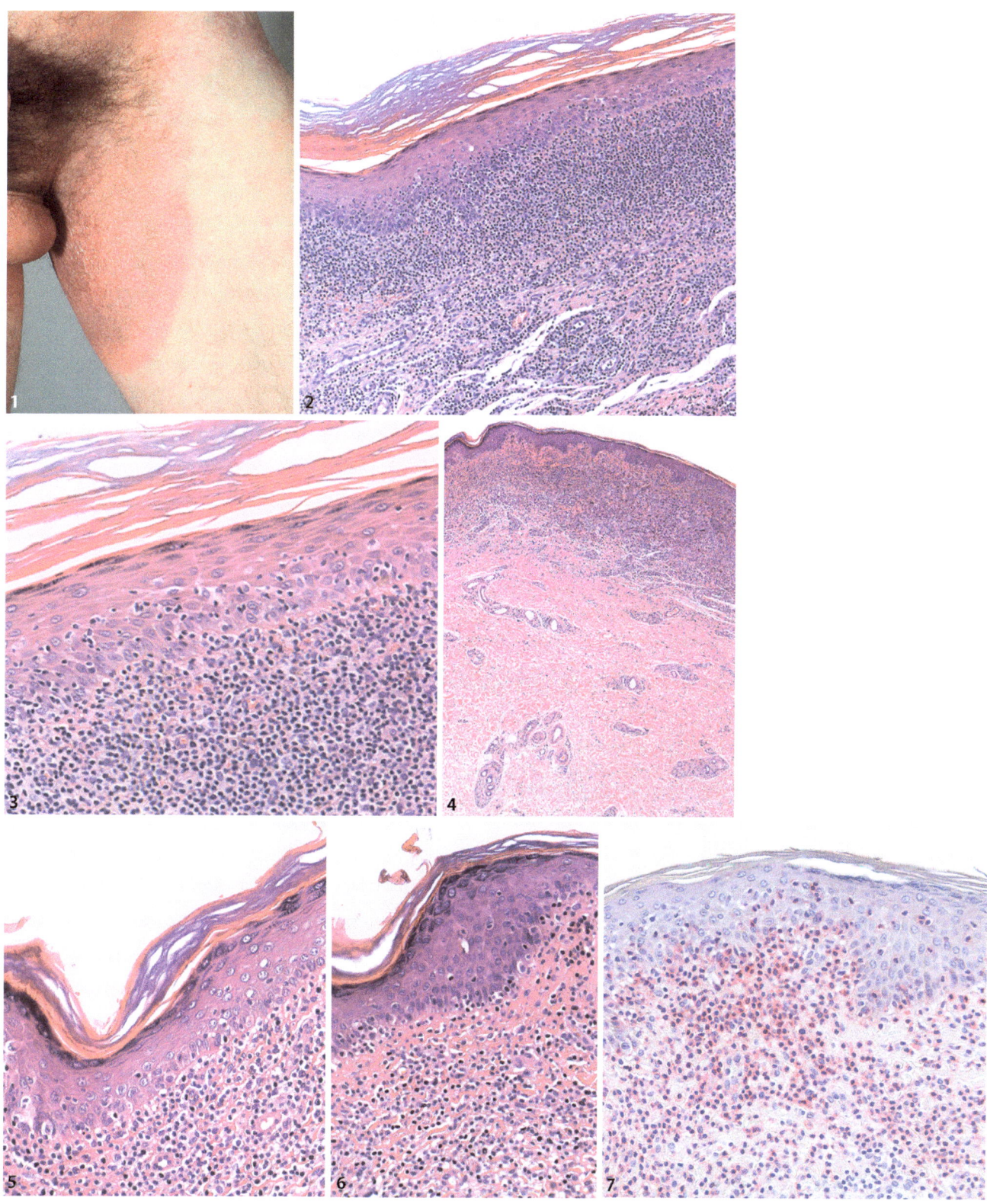

Primary cutaneous pleomorphic small/medium-sized T-cell lymphoma revealed by a plantar callus

G. Quereux and B. Dreno

Age: 54 years   **Sex:** M

Clinical features: Isolated hyperkeratosic lesion of 2 cm of diameter, painless, on the heel, onset 2 years before, with an aspect of an ordinary callus. Central crack appeared as the lesion increased in size. The histology found, under an hyperkeratosic epidermis a dermal infiltrate constituted of medium-sized lymphoid elements with occasional notched nucleus, without epidermotropism; the lymphocytes were CD3+ CD8+ CD30–. The PCR revealed a clonal T-cell population in the biopsy.

Diagnosis: Primary cutaneous pleomorphic small/medium-sized T-cell lymphoma (PSMTCL).

Follow-up: CT-scan (chest and abdominal), abdomino-pelvic ultrasonography and bone marrow biopsy were negative. As the lesion was isolated, surgical excision was decided. It was supplemented with a radiotherapy of 20 Grays due to some remaining tumoral lesion. Seven months later the patient was still in complete clinical remission.

Comment: PSMTCL is a rare, recently recognized type of cutaneous T cell lymphoma (CTCL), representing about 3% of all primary CTCLs. Onset ranges from 50 to 60 years of age. Clinically, PSMTCL is different from the mycosis fongoide (MF). It is characterized by one or more red-purple papulo-nodules, tumours often ulcerated, or deeply infiltrated plaques, on the trunk and extremities, and by the absence of pruritus and preexistent lesions.

Histologically, it is characterized by rare epidermotropism, a major dermal infiltrate frequently involving the subcutaneous tissue. This dense, nodular or diffuse infiltrate, is composed of lymphoid cells of small to medium-sized pleomorphic lymphocytes with irregular, but not cerebriform nuclei. By definition large pleomorphic cells are present in less than 30% in the infiltrate. The majority of tumour cells in PSMTCL are CD4+, CD8–, with frequent loss of pan-T antigens. The T-cell receptor gene analysis in the skin confirms the presence of monoclonal lymphocytes. According to the few cases reported in the literature, the prognosis of PSMTCL seems good.

Our case is interesting because of its clinical originality: indeed, the hyperkeratosic form of PSMTLC has never been reported in the literature.

- **Fig. 1:** Hyperkeratosic lesion on the heel mimicking an ordinary callus.
- **Fig. 2:** Closer view of the lesion.

References

Friedmann D, Wechsler J, Delfau MH, Esteve E, Farcet JP, of Low wall A, Parneix-Spake A, Valiant L, Revuz J, Bagot M (1995) Primary cutaneous pleomorphic small T-cell lymphoma. With review of 11 boxes. The French Group Study one Cutaneous Lymphomas. Arch Dermatol 131:1009–1015

Kim YC, Vandersteen DP (2001) Primary cutaneous pleomorphic small/medium-sized T-cell lymphoma in a young man. Br J Dermatol. 144:903–905

Von den Driesch P, Coors EA. Localized cutaneous small to medium-sized pleomorphic T-cell lymphoma: a report of 3 cases stable for years (2002) J Am Acad Dermatol 46:531–535

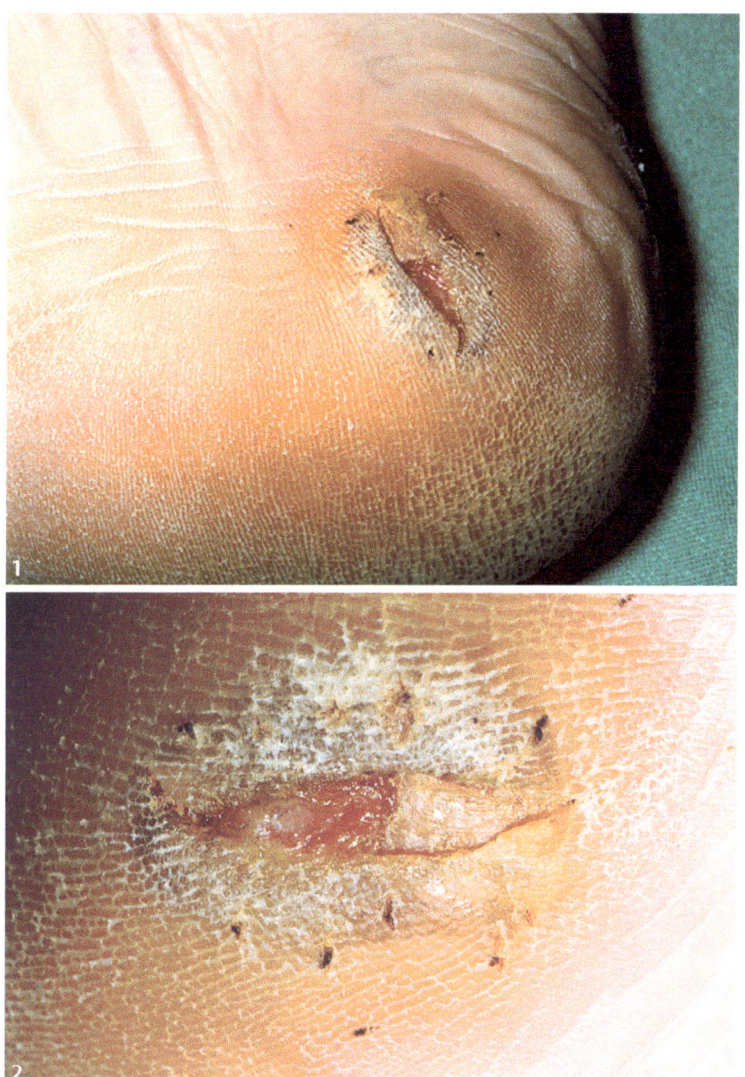

Atypical poorly differentiated cutaneous T-cell lymphoma with an angiocentric growth pattern

B. Laetsch and R. Dummer

Age: 41 years   **Sex:** M

Clinical features: Infiltrated and ulcerated circular skin lesions were for over two years restricted to the legs. At a later date they spread to arms and trunk and the patient presented with generalized hyperpigmentation, pruritus and multiple ulcerations as well as generalized alopecia. Lymph nodes were enlarged. Biopsies of early lesions showed lymphocytic vasculitis, later there was a diffuse infiltrate of medium-sized to large pleomorphic cells with irregular nuclei. The vast majority of these cells expressed CD4, but only about 50% CD3. Genomic DNA was amplified by polymerase chain reaction using primers for $V\gamma$ 1–11 and $J\gamma$ 1/2 as well as $JP\gamma$ 1/2. Using primers $V\gamma$ 10,11 and J1/2 a clonal population was detected in the fourth skin biopsy and in the peripheral blood. Sequencing revealed the same rearrangement of the V10 and J2 segment of the TCR γ in the skin biopsy as well as in the blood.

Diagnosis: Atypical poorly differentiated cutaneous T-cell lymphoma with an angiocentric growth pattern.

Follow-up: The patient did not respond to various therapeutic attempts (CHOP chemotherapy, topic and systemic steroids, extracorporeal photopheresis and Interferon-a-therapy) The disease progressed: with erythroderma, massive exfoliation and numerous ulcers with a diameter of up to 5 cm on arms and legs. The patient died very soon.

Comment: Initially the skin lesions were clinically and histologically diagnosed as vasculitis. Only later the diagnosis of a T-Cell lymphoma could have been established histologically and with the aid of molecular biologic analysis. The tumor cells showed an angiocentric growth pattern but didn't express CD3 nor CD 56 which is atypical for this subtype of lymphoma. Few cases of cutaneous angiocentric lymphomas are reported without CD56 but with CD3 expression. Theses patients presented with leg lesions as first manifestation of the neoplasm as well similar to our patient. As the early detected neoplastic clonal cells in the peripheral blood were of small cell convoluted type and the neoplastic infiltrating cell in the skin biopsy where large cell blastoid cells that expressed only the panleukocyte marker CD45RO, we assume that there was a transformation into a more undifferentiated and aggressive lymphoma type.

Fig. 1: Multiple ulcerations on the trunk.

Fig. 2: Closer view of the lesions on the leg.

Fig. 3: Diffuse, dense infiltrate in all dermal layers.The infiltrate is perivascularly accentuated. Microscopic magnification 250×.

Fig. 4: The infiltrate consists of granulocytes, histiocytes and large blastoid cell. Focally atypical mitoses can be seen. Microscopic magnification 400×.

Fig. 5: CD3 staining. About 50% of the tumour cells show positivity. Microscopic magnification 250×.

References

Cho K, Kim C, Yang S, Kim B, Kim J (1997) Angiocentric T cell lymphoma of the skin presenting as inflammatory nodules of the leg. Clinical & Experimental Dermatology 22:104–108

Meyer JC, Hassam S, Dummer R, Muletta S, Dobbeling U, Dommann SN, Burg G (1997) A realistic approach to the sensitivity of PCR-DGGE and its application as a sensitive tool for the detection of clonality in cutaneous T-cell proliferations. Experimental Dermatology 6:122–127

Niitsu N, Umeda M (1996) Angiocentric T cell lymphoma with prominent cutaneous ulceration. Leukemia 10:1249–1251

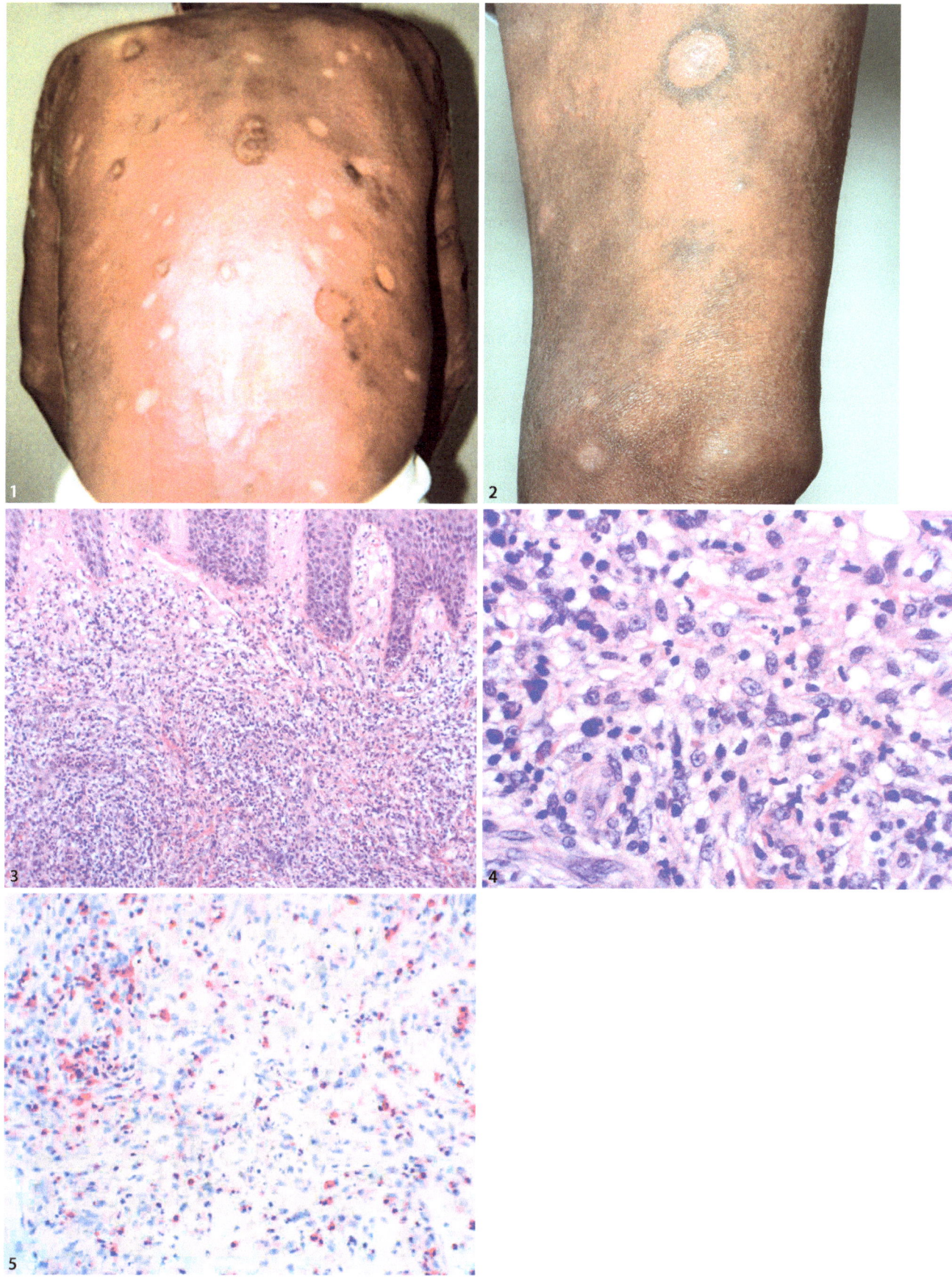

Angiocentric non-Hodgkin's lymphoma of the leg

G. S. WOOD and M. A. HINSHAW

Age: 30 years   **Sex:** F

Clinical Features: Eleven-year history of a large, progessive ulceration of the right lower extremity. A smaller but similar lesion on the left ankle was excised approximately 15 years prior. No clinical follow-up from that lesion was done.

Diagnosis: Angiocentric non-Hodgkin's lymphoma of the leg.

Follow-up: Required above-knee amputation for refractory disease.

Comment: Angiocentric lymphoma is a CD30-negative non-mycosis fungoides primary cutaneous T-cell lymphoma according to the EORTC classification system. Typical presentation is with nodules and plaques often on the lower extremities that may ulcerate. Systemic symptoms such as fever malaise, and weight loss are not uncommon. Further classifying these lymphomas has not correlated with prognosis. Clonal rearrangements of T-cell receptor genes are present in a subset of cases. In our patient, multiple fungal, bacterial, and atypical mycobacterial cultures were negative. PPD and HIV tests were negative. Chest, abdomen, and pelvic computerized tomogaphy did not show evidence of systemic involvement.

The infiltrate is composed of pleomorphic lymphocytes with large, irregularly shaped, densely chromatic nuclei. Cytology may be either large or small/medium lymphocytes. Epidermotropism may or may not be present. An angiocentric lymphoid infiltrate may extend into the subcutaneous fat or occasionally have a peri-adnexal distribution with adnexal destruction. In general, scattered plasma cells and histiocytes, with occasional granulomas are typical. Characteristic findings include lymphocytic vasculitis with endothelial swelling, fibrin deposition in vascular wall and lumina, and an onion skin-like proliferation of the vascular wall. Our patient's T-cell infiltrate was CD2+, CD4+ and variably deficient in CD3, CD5 and CD7. PCR/DGGE was polyclonal.

The clinical course is marked by dissemination with hepatosplenomegaly and bone marrow involvement. Interestingly, peripheral lymph nodes are usually spared, especially in early stages of the disease. Our patient's case is unusual due to the prolonged disease course and lack of systemic involvement.

Treatment may include multi-agent chemotherapy with or without prednisone, interferon-alpha (IFNa), and external beam radiation therapy. Unfortunately, our patient's disease was refractory to each of these treatments. She required above-knee amputation for progressive disease but is currently free of lymphoma.

- **Fig. 1:** Right lateral leg showing chronic ulceration and scar.
- **Fig. 2:** Ulcerated tumor in various stages of evolution.
- **Fig. 3:** A pan-dermal, pleomorphic, lymphocytic infiltrate is angiocentric and extends into the subcutaneous tissue.
- **Fig. 4:** The angiocentric, angiodestructive nature of the tumor is depicted here.
- **Fig. 5:** Pleomorphic tumor cells with numerous mitoses in this high power field.
- **Fig. 6: a** Semi-serial sections showing a high proportion of CD2+ cells. **b** CD5 stains a smaller proportion of these cells.

References

El Shabrawi-Caelen L, Cerroni L, Kerl H (2000) The clinicopathologic spectrum of cytotoxic lymphomas of the skin. Sem Cut Med & Surg 19:118–123

Gilliam AC, Wood GS (199) Primary cutaneous lymphomas other than mycosis fungoides. Sem Oncol 26:290–306

Harris N, Jaffe E, Stein H et al. (1994) A revised European-American classification of lymphoid neoplasms: A proposal from the International Lymphoma Study Group. Blood 84:1361–1392

Willemze R (2000) Primary cutaneous lymphomas. Curr Opin in Onc 12:419–425

Willemze R, Kerl H, Sterry W et al. (1997) EORTC Classification for primary cutaneous lymphomas: A proposal from the cutaneous lymphoma study group of the European organization for research and treatment of cancer. Blood 90:354–371

Wood GS (2001) The Benign and Malignant Cutaneous Lymphoproliferative disorders including mycosis fungoides. Neoplastic Hematopathology. 2nd Ed. D.M. Knowles (ed), Baltimore, MD: Williams and Wilkins, 1183–1233

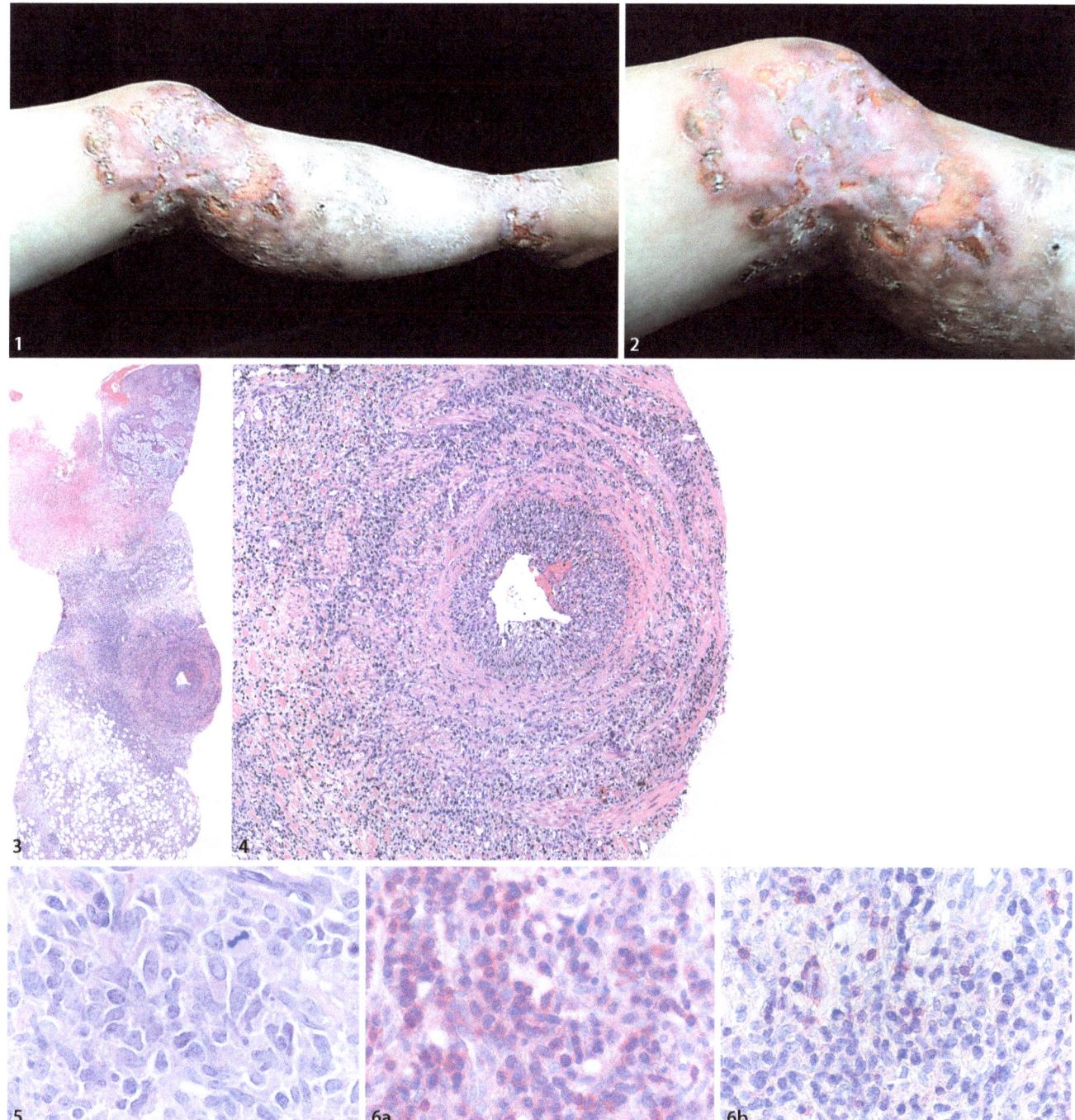

■ γ/δ cutaneous T-cell lymphoma

R. H. Weenig and L. E. Gibson

Age: 63 years   **Sex:** M

Clinical Features: Six-month history of multiple purple indurated papules and subcutaneous nodules involving the thighs, trunk and forehead, and an edematous ulcerated left leg. Staging work-up was negative.

TCR gene analysis: T-cell clone detected using Southern-Blot analysis (Eco R-1 digest of J-region of gamma-chain).

Diagnosis: Primary cutaneous γ/δ T-cell lymphoma.

Follow-up: The patient died 17 months after diagnosis, cause of death unknown.

Comment: Gamma/delta cutaneous T-cell lymphoma (GDCTCL) has been considered by many to be a variant of subcutaneous panniculitis-like T-cell lymphoma (SPTCL). Recent work (Massone et al. 2004 and Toro et al. 2003) suggests that GDCTCL is a distinct clinicopathologic entity based on phenotypic differences and an aggressive clinical course. GDCTCL usually is associated with dermal and/or epidermal involvement by neoplastic lymphocytes in addition to the subcutaneous involvement typified by SPTCL. The immunophenotype of the neoplastic lymphocytes in cases of GDCTCL are as follows: positive for CD2, CD3, TIA-1, and Granzyme B; variably positive for CD5, CD7, and CD56; and negative for CD4, CD8, and BF-1. Distinction from nasal type extranodal NK/T-cell lymphoma is made by identification of a CD3-surface expression and a positive T-cell receptor gene rearrangement in GDCTCL.

- ▦ **Fig. 1:** Patchy nodular dermal and diffuse lobular pannicular lymphoid infiltrate. Microscopic magnification 25×.
- ▦ **Fig. 2:** Diffuse lobular lymphoid infiltrate. Microscopic magnification 50×.
- ▦ **Fig. 3:** Small – medium sized pleomorphic lymphoid cells. Microscopic magnification 400×.
- ▦ **Fig. 4:** CD2 positive staining. Microscopic magnification 100×.
- ▦ **Fig. 5:** CD3 positive staining. Microscopic magnification 100×.
- ▦ **Fig. 6:** CD8 negative staining. Microscopic magnification 200×.
- ▦ **Fig. 7:** BF-1 negative staining. Microscopic magnification 100×.
- ▦ **Fig. 8:** Granzyme-B positive staining. Microscopic magnification 100×.

References

Massone C, Chott A, Metze D et al. (2004) Subcutaneous, blastic natural killer (NK), NK/T-cell, and other cytotoxic lymphomas of the skin: a morphologic, immunophenotypic, and molecular study of 50 patients. Am J Surg Pathol 28:719–735

Toro JR, Liewehr DJ, Pabby N et al. (2003) Gamma-delta T-cell phenotype is associated with significantly decreased survival in cutaneous T-cell lymphoma. Blood 101:3407–3412

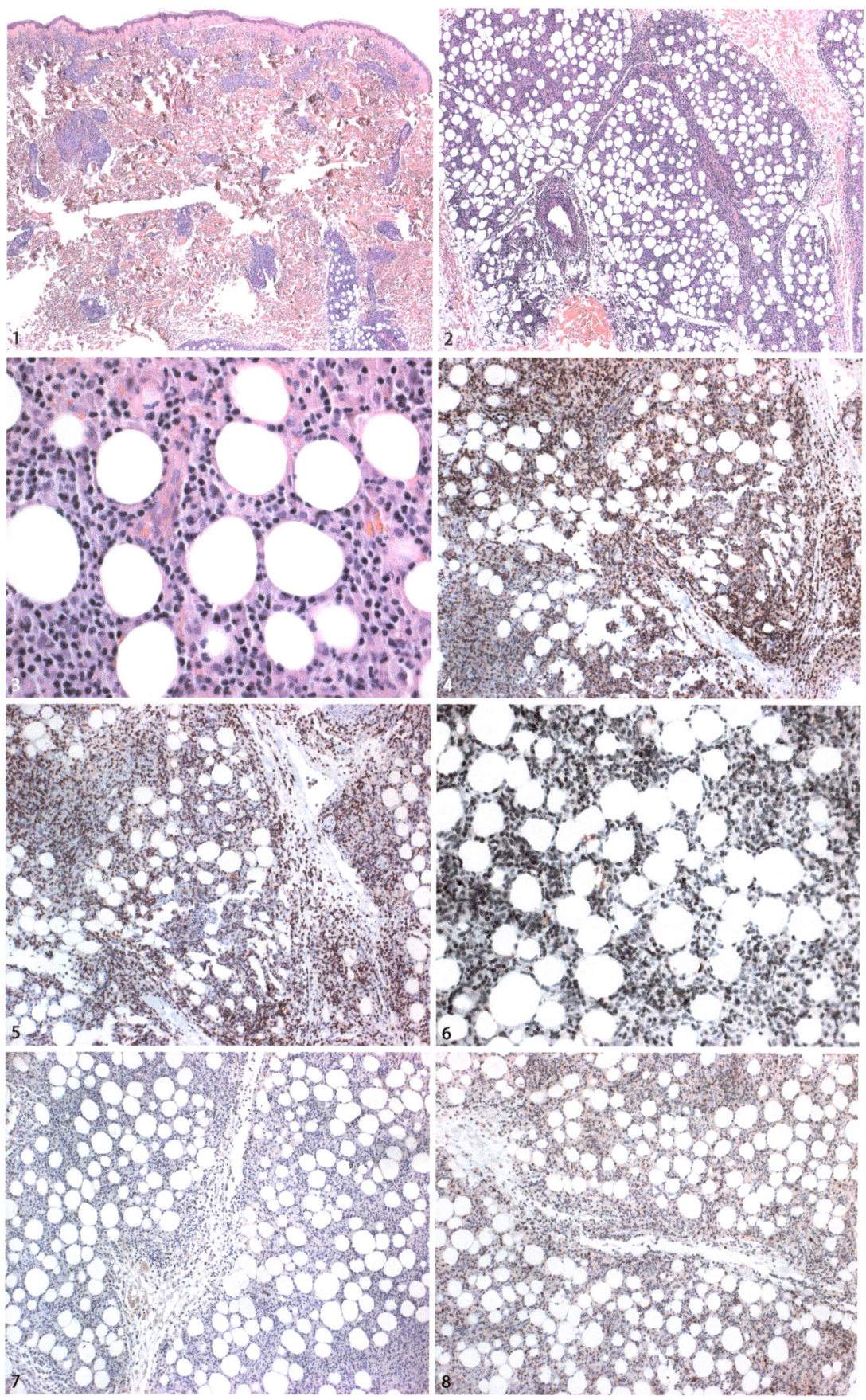

■ Epidermotropic and subcutaneous γ/δ T-cell lymphoma

L. Cerroni and H. Kerl

Age: 34 years **Sex:** M

Clinical features: Multiple reddish, partly infiltrated, partly slightly erosive plaques and subcutaneous tumors on the trunk and extremities with involvement of the conjunctiva and of the oral mucosa. The skin lesions were present for the last 2 months. The patient had also general symptoms (fever, malaise).

Diagnosis: Cutaneous γ/δ T-cell lymphoma with epidermotropic and subcutaneous involvement.

Follow-up: The patient died within a few weeks.

Comment: Cutaneous γ/δ T-cell lymphoma is a rare subtype of the cutaneous T-cell lymphomas (CTCLs) with aggressive behaviour and poor prognosis. Distinction between primary and secondary cutaneous involvement in these cases is of limited importance, and bears little, if any, prognostic value. Cutaneous lesions are characterized by involvement of the epidermis with marked epidermotropism and/or of the subcutaneous fat tissue, simulating the picture of mycosis fungoides and of subcutaneous T-cell lymphoma, respectively. Most patients will show both patterns either at the same time (even in the same biopsy) or in biopsies taken at different times. Differentiation from subcutaneous T-cell lymphoma can be achieved upon careful phenotypic investigations: subcutaneous T-cell lymphoma is characterized by a $\gamma/\delta-$, CD8+ phenotype of neoplastic cells, in contrast to the $\gamma/\delta+$ phenotype of cutaneous γ/δ T-cell lymphoma. Differentiation from mycosis fungoides can be achieved only upon correlation with the clinical features: in fact, cutaneous T-cell lymphoma shows ulcerated plaques and tumors at onset, whereas mycosis fungoides slowly progresses over years or decades through the well-known patch-, plaque- and tumor-stages. In many instances patients with cutaneous γ/δ T-cell lymphoma present clinical features of haemophagocytic syndrome, which is often the cause of death in these patients.

▦ **Fig. 1:** Multiple reddish, partly subcutaneous, partly erosive plaques and tumors on the trunk.

▦ **Fig. 2:** Histopathologic features of two biopsies taken at different sites on the same day. Superficial infiltrate with marked epidermotropism (a) and prominent infiltrate of the subcutaneous fat tissues (b).

▦ **Fig. 3:** Detail of the superficial infiltrate with marked epidermotropism.

▦ **Fig. 4:** Positivity of neoplastic cells for CD56.

References

Cerroni L, Gatter K, Kerl H (2004) An illustrated guide to skin lymphoma. 2nd edition. Malden, Oxford, Carlton, Blackwell Publishing

Massone C, Chott A, Metze D et al. (2004) Subcutaneous, blastic natural killer (NK), NK/T-cell, and other cytotoxic lymphomas of the skin. A morphologic, immunophenotypic, and molecular study of 50 patients. Am J Surg Pathol 28:719–735

Munn SE, McGregor JM, Jones A et al. (1996) Clinical and pathological heterogeneity in cutaneous gamma-delta T-cell lymphoma: a report of three cases and a review of the literature. Br J Dermatol 135:976–981

Toro JR, Liewehr DJ, Pabby N (2003) Gamma-delta T-cell phenotype is associated with significantly decreased survival in cutaneous T-cell lymphoma. Blood 101: 3407–3412

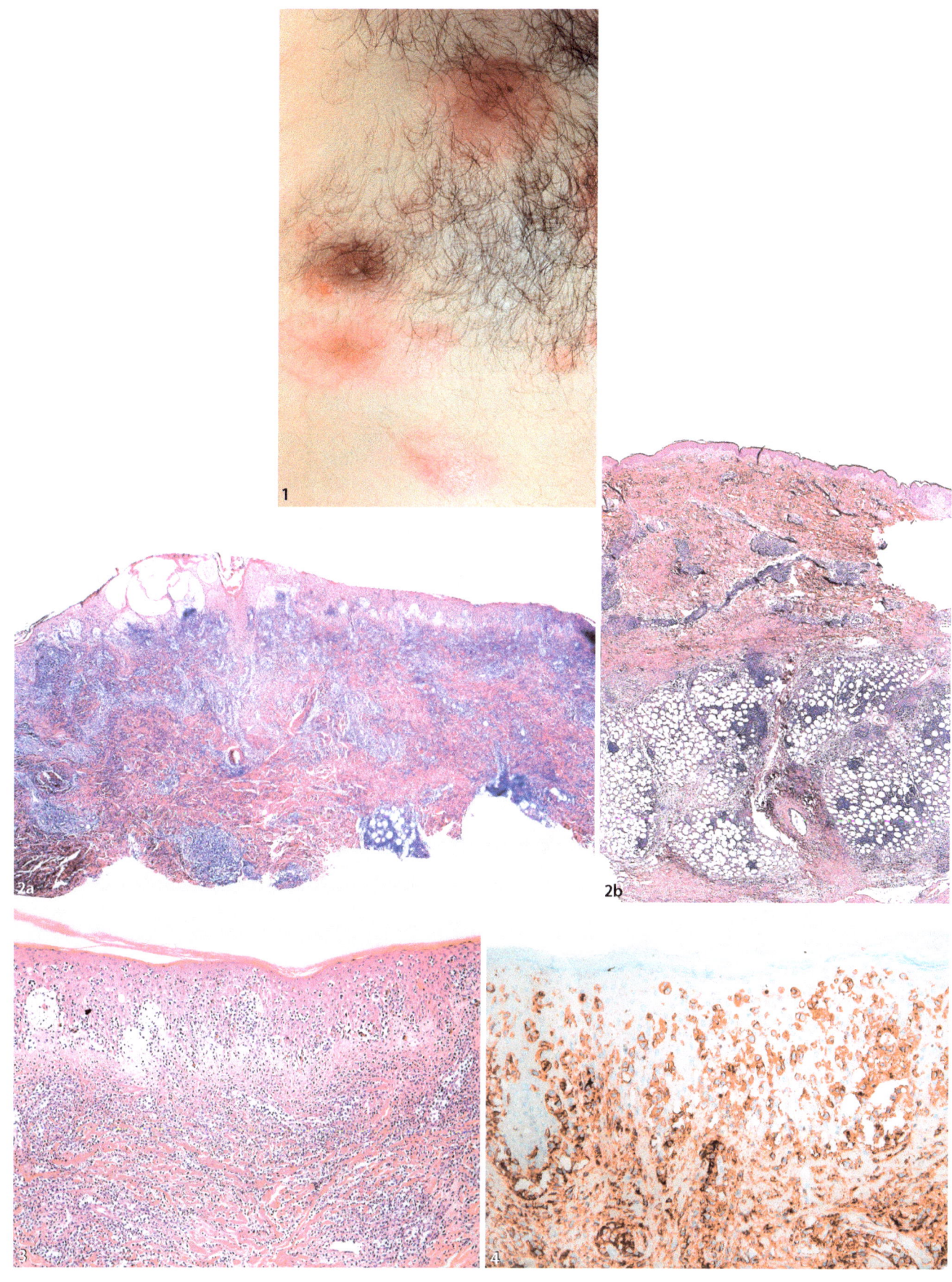

Cutaneous T-cell lymphoma presenting as reticular erythematous mucinosis

J. M. TWERSKY and D. F. MUTASIM

CASE a

Age: 66 years   **Sex:** M

Clinical features: A 66-year-old white man presented with a six-month history of an asymptomatic reticulated erythematous macular eruption on the back and chest that was clinically consistent with reticular erythematous mucinosis (REM). Histologic examination revealed a mild to moderate superficial perivascular and perifollicular lymphocytic infiltrate with epidermotropism of single and grouped lymphocytes. The lymphocytic infiltrate was insufficient to perform immunophenotyping on the specimen. A leukocyte dehydrogenase level and a complete blood count with differential were within normal limits. HTLV-1 antibody testing was negative. A blood smear preparation revealed that 24% of the circulating lymphocytes had convoluted nuclei. PCR analysis revealed a monoclonal T-cell receptor gamma gene rearrangement in the patient's blood, indicating the presence of a circulating monoclonal T-cell population. Flow cytometric analysis of bone marrow aspirate and biopsy material were unremarkable. CT scan of the chest, abdomen and pelvis was negative.

Diagnosis: Cutaneous T-cell lymphoma, mycosis fungoides (MF) type, mimicking reticular erythematous mucinosis.

Follow-up: The patient's condition remained unchanged at 18 months after presentation.

Comment: The above case of CTCL clinically simulated REM, a novel clinical presentation of CTCL. Involvement of extracutaneous sites (within six months) occurred early. This observation suggests that the atypical presentation of CTCL mimicking REM may be more aggressive than typical patch-stage disease in which mortality is not significantly different from matched controls.

This variant of CTCL clinically mimicking REM should be added to the multiple clinical presentations already reported. This clinical presentation of CTCL emphasizes the protean manifestations of the disease and the need for careful clinical observation and appropriate histologic analysis of cases suspected of having REM. Patients with CTCL simulating REM should be carefully evaluated at presentation for extracutaneous disease and should be closely monitored for more rapid progression to systemic involvement.

- **Fig. 1:** Reticulated, smooth, erythematous patches over the upper back and neck.
- **Fig. 2:** Closer view of figure 1.
- **Fig. 3:** Increased amount of mucin in the dermis. Inset with epidermotropic infiltrate.

References

Fung MA, Murphy MJ, Hoss DM et al. (2002) Practical evaluation and management of cutaneous lymphoma. J Am Acad Dermatol 46:25–57; quiz, 358–360

Kim YH, Jensen RA, Watanabe GL et al. (1996) Clinical stage IA (limited patch and plaque) mycosis fungoides. A long-term outcome analysis. Arch Dermatol 132:1309–1313

Twersky JM, Mutasim DF: Mycosis Fungoides Presenting as Reticular Erythematous Mucinosis. Int J Dermatol (In press)

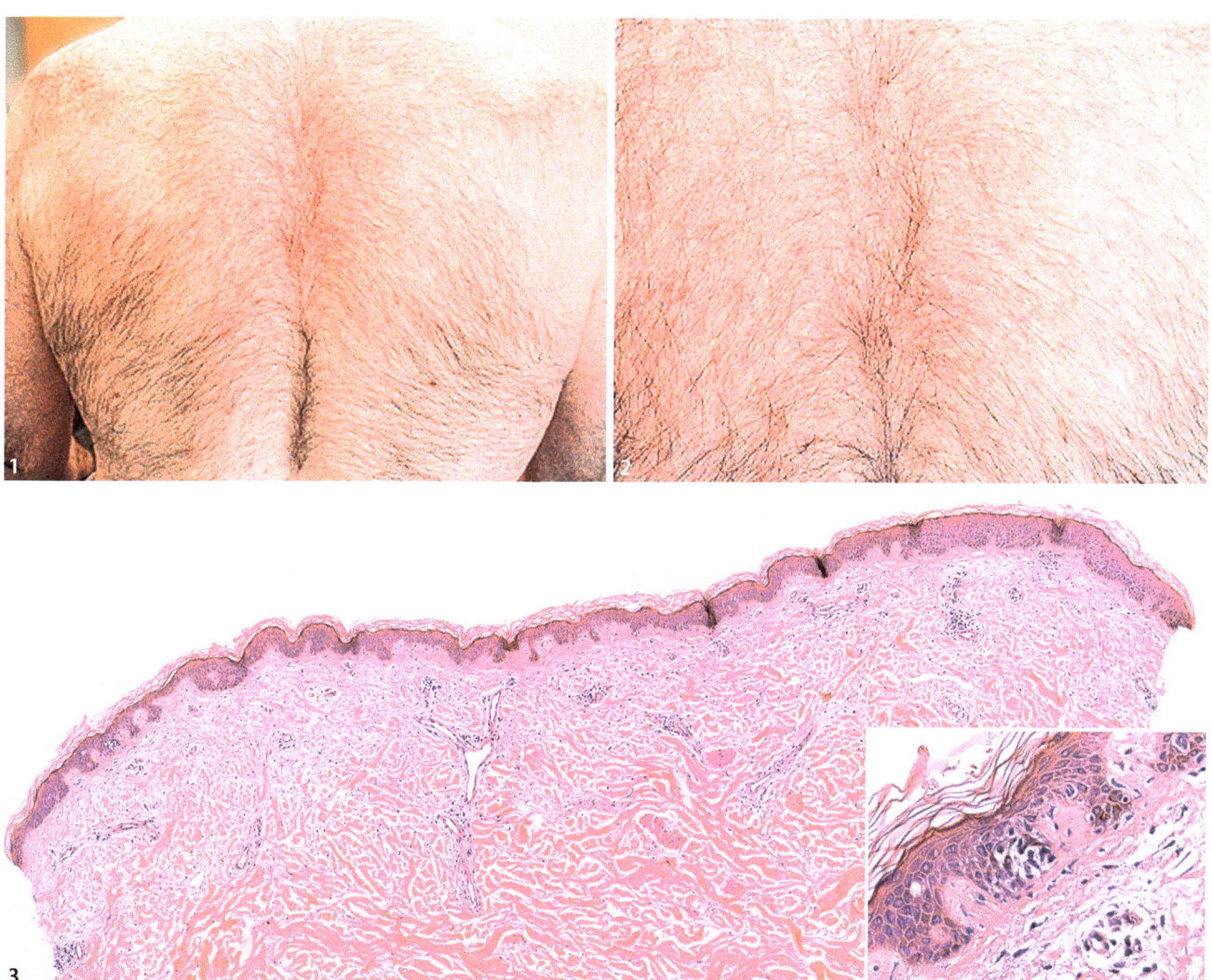

CASE b

Age: 50 years   **Sex:** M

Clinical features: Mildly pruritic, reticulated erythematous smooth patches that worsened in the summer on the chest, back, arms and face first appeared in 1994 at 48 years of age. Based on clinicopathologic correlation, a diagnosis of reticular erythematous mucinosis (REM) was made.

The patient was unresponsive to therapy including mid-potency steroid ointments, UVB, and hydroxychloroquine over a subsequent three-year period. Repeat histologic examination revealed findings of CTCL. At this time, immunophenotyping of the infiltrate revealed 80–90% of the lymphocytes to be CD4+ with an elevated CD4/CD8 ratio (14.5, normal 2:1) and marked loss of CD7 staining (less than 10% CD7+). White blood cell count was normal (8,400/ml) with 54% lymphocytes. No clonality was found in the circulating lymphocytes by T-cell receptor gene rearrangement. Antibodies to HTLV-1 were not detected. CT scans of chest, abdomen, and pelvis revealed no systemic involvement. The patient's disease continued to progress.

At age 56, repeat evaluation revealed a leukocytosis of 17,900/ml with 67% lymphocytes and 15% atypical lymphocytes with convoluted nuclei. Flow cytometry studies of peripheral blood and bone marrow aspirate revealed a homogeneous population of CD4+, CD7-, and CD29+ lymphocytes in both specimens. The CD4/CD8 ratio was markedly elevated (18:1 in the peripheral blood and 14.5 in the bone marrow). LDH level was normal and CT scans of the chest, abdomen and pelvis were unremarkable.

Diagnosis: Stage IVB cutaneous CD4+ T-cell lymphoma (CTCL) which initially mimicked reticular erythematous mucinosis.

Follow-up: After two years of successful control using mid-potency corticosteroid ointments, prednisone and chlorambucil, the patient's disease progressed to plaques and tumors. Multiple therapies were ineffective, including topical mechlorethamine, photochemotherapy, methotrexate, gemcitabine, intravenous pentostatin, and total skin electron beam radiation followed by oral bexarotene. Eight years after initial presentation, the patient developed a rapidly declining course with erythroderma, respiratory failure, disseminated intravascular coagulation, and acute renal failure eventuating in death due to multiorgan failure.

Comment: CTCL clinically simulating REM is rare, but it may have a more progressive course. This patient was treated for REM unsuccessfully for three years before studies revealed a diagnosis of CTCL which eventually had a fatal course. Of note, the peripheral blood gene rearrangement studies revealed no monoclonal population, even when repeated in the advanced stage. False negative results may occur due to sample size, sampling error, and other technical limitations.

Based on the early involvement of extracutaneous sites (within six years) and the fatal outcome within eight years of initial presentation, the course of this patient is more aggressive than would be predicted by the presentation with patch-stage disease. Additionally, the lack of response to multiple topical and systemic lymphoma therapies suggests a more resistant form of CTCL. These observations suggest that the atypical presentation of CTCL mimicking REM may be more aggressive than typical patch-stage disease in which mortality is not significantly different from matched controls.

■ **Fig. 1:** Reticulated, smooth, erythematous patches over the upper chest and neck (**a**). Closer view of Figure 1a (**b**).

■ **Fig. 2:** There were several Pautrier's microabscesses containing hyperchromatic lymphocytes with halos and a dense superficial lymphocytic infiltrate, characteristic of MF. HE, microscopic magnification 150×).

■ **Fig. 3:** Indurated plaques in a generalized distribution (**a**). Closer view of Figure 3a (**b**).

■ **Fig. 4:** Centrally ulcerated tumor on the left thigh.

■ **Fig. 5:** Erythroderma.

References

Fung MA, Murphy MJ, Hoss DM et al. (2002) Practical evaluation and management of cutaneous lymphoma. J Am Acad Dermatol 46: 325-57; quiz, 358–360

Zackheim HS, Amin S, Kashani-Sabet M et al. (1999) Prognosis in cutaneous T-cell lymphoma by skin stage: long-term survival in 489 patients. J Am Acad Dermatol 40: 418–425

Twersky JM, Mutasim DF: Mycosis Fungoides Presenting as Reticular Erythematous Mucinosis. Int J Dermatol (in press)

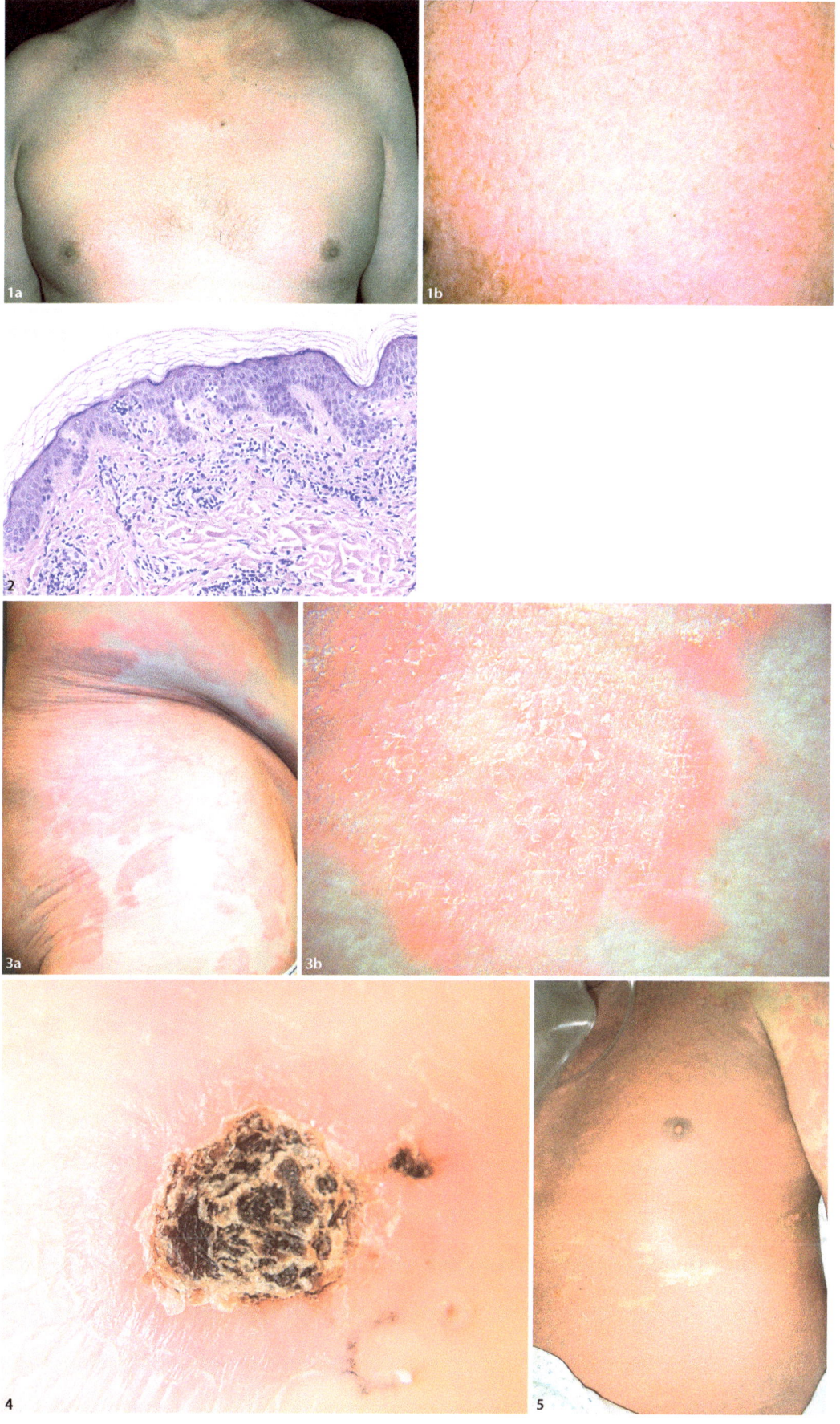

■ Nasal NK-cell lymphoma preceded by a puffy eyelid and swollen cheek due to intramuscular infiltration of Epstein-Barr virus-infected cells

K. IWATSUKI and M. OHTSUKA

Age: 16 years   **Sex:** M

Clinical features: The patient had repetitive swelling of the right cheek since 10 years old, which resolved spontaneously. At the age of 16 years, asymptomatic puffy swelling occurred on the left eyelid associated with the right cheek swelling. No systemic symptoms or other cutaneous manifestations were observed. The following laboratory test results were normal or negative: complete blood cell counts, blood chemistry, and urinalysis. The percentages of NK cells (CD2+/56+) in the peripheral blood ranged from 14–16%. The antibody titers to EB virus were as follows: anti-VCA IgG, 1:1280; anti-VCA IgA, 1:80; anti-EA IgG, 1:640; anti-EA IgA, 1:40; and anti-EBNA, 1:20. Intramuscular infiltration of NK/T cells together with a considerable number of EBER-positive cells was present in the eyelid and cheek.

Diagnosis: EB virus-associated NK cell lymphoproliferative disorder with malignant potential.

Follow-up: He was treated with IFN-γ 2 million units intravenously five times per week, but the swelling of the eyelid and cheek was not resolved. Two years later, he presented with nasal obstruction and fever. Biopsy specimens from the nasal cavity showed the feature of nasal lymphoma with infiltration of tumor cells positive for CD3ε, CD56, TIA-1 and granzyme B, and negative for CD4, CD8, and CD20. His hard and soft palates were perforated due to the infiltration of the tumor cells. Despite the polychemotherapy followed by autologous peripheral blood stem cell transplantation, he died of the progression of the illness.

Comment: The patient had persistent but non-progressive swelling of the eyelid and cheek with the infiltration of NK/T cells carrying a latent EB virus infection for at least 9 years. A puffy eyelid or cheek swelling might be a unique cutaneous manifestation preceded by the occurrence of overt EB virus-associated NK/T cell lymphomas. In addition to the diagnostic tests such as the detection of EBV-infected NK/T cells and the measurement of anti-EB virus antibody titers, the monitoring of EBV DNA load in the blood might be useful to predict the progression of nasal NK cell lymphoma.

- **Fig. 1:** Swelling of the left eyelid at the age of 16 (the same patient described in Br J Dermatol 1999, Ohtsuka M et al).
- **Fig. 2:** Swelling of the right cheek at the age of 16.
- **Fig. 3:** Lymphocytic infiltration into the muscle (buccinator muscle).
- **Fig. 4:** Medium-sized lymphoid cells are present between muscle bundles.
- **Fig. 5:** A considerable number of EB virus-encoded small nuclear RNA (EBER)-positive cells are present in the infiltrates.
- **Fig. 6:** CD56-positive cells are infiltrated.
- **Fig. 7:** Cells expressing cytotoxic molecules are present in the infiltrates (Fig.: Granzyme B).
- **Fig. 8:** The soft and hard palates are perforated due to the infiltration of the tumor cells.
- **Fig. 9:** An infiltrative shadow is observed in the right maxillary sinus.

References

Ohtsuka M, Iwatsuki K, Kaneko R et al. (1999) Epstein-Barr virus-associated lymphoid hyperplasia of the eyelid characterized by intramuscular infiltration. Br J Dermatol 140:358–377

Shirasaki F, Taniuchi K, Matsushita T et al. (2002) Epstein-Barr virus-associated T-cell lymphoma: a case of eyelid swelling and intramuscular infiltration mimicking dermatomyositis. Br J Dermatol 147:1244–1248

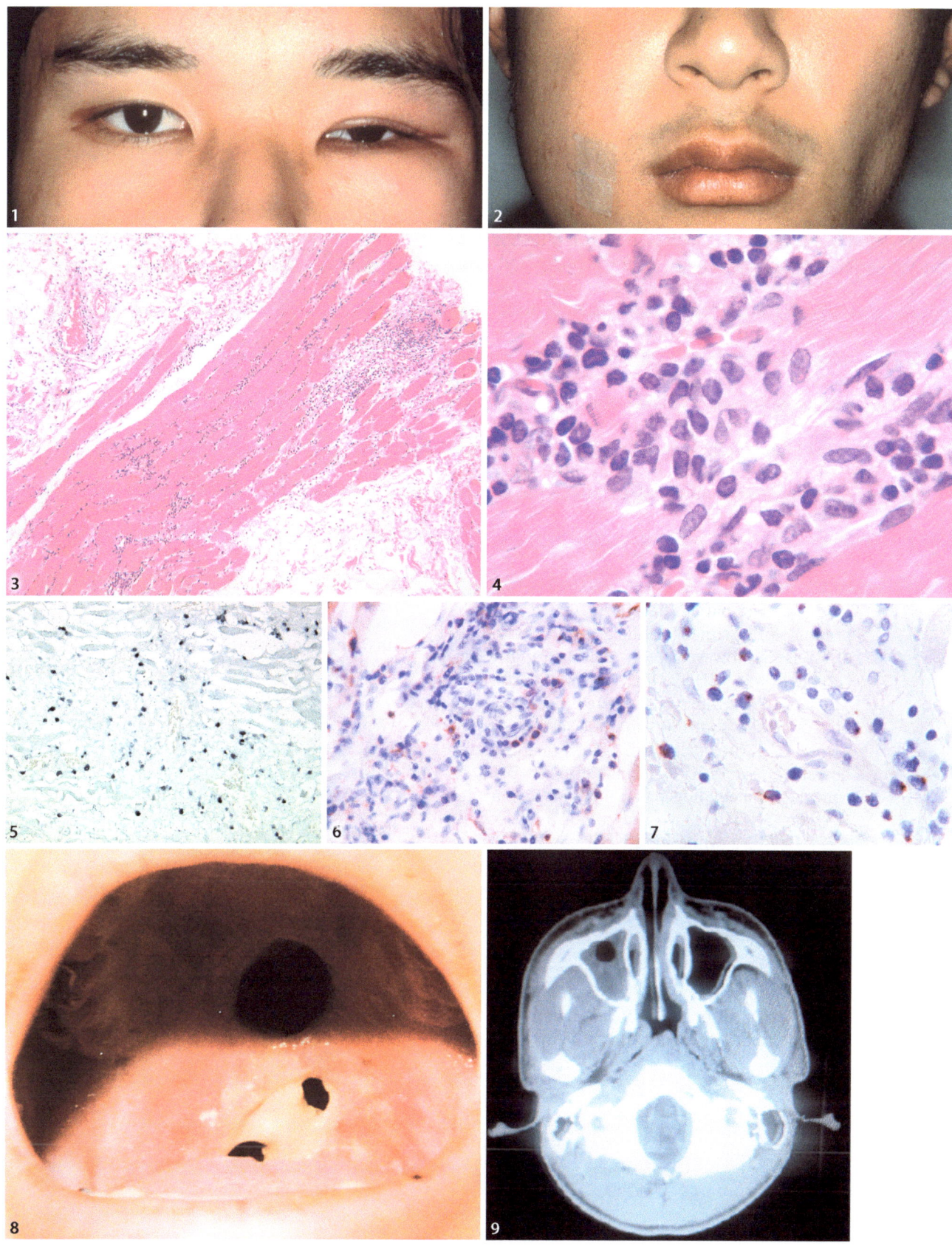

Epstein-Barr virus-associated lymphoma mimicking hydroa vacciniforme: Final diagnosis of a case reported in 1986

T. Oono

Age: 16 years   **Sex:** M

Clinical features: At the age of 6 years, he began to have recurrent vesicles on the sun-exposed areas in summer. At the age of 14 years, recurrent edema of the face began to develop. After admission, he developed headache, general malaise and high-fever. Cervical lymph nodes were swollen. Histopathological findings of a vesicle were compatible with hydroa vacciniforme (HV). A cervical lymph node specimen showed destruction of original architecture with infiltration of atypical lymphocytes with numerous mitoses. The patient was diagnosed as having HV and malignant lymphoma in 1986.

Diagnosis: Coexistence of HV and malignant lymphoma (T cell).

Follow-up: The patient had been treated with oral prednisolone with a beneficial effect. At the age of 18 years, however, liver function rapidly exacerbated, and CHOP therapy was performed. The laboratory findings indicated those of hemophagocytosis, showing aspartate aminotransferase; 66 IU/L (normal; 9 to 27 IU/L), alanine aminotransferase; 45 IU/L(normal; 6 to 37 IU/L), serum lactic dehydrogenase; 1418 IU/L (normal; 111 to 377 IU/L), a red blood cell count; $4.72 \times 10^6/\mu l$, a white blood cell count; $1.8 \times 10^3/\mu l$, a platelet count; $64 \times 10^3/\mu l$. The patient died of disseminated actinomycosis. Autopsy findings revealed fatal hemophagocytosis in lymph nodes, spleen, bone marrow and liver.

Comment: The role of Epstein-Barr virus (EBV) in the pathogenesis of HV is recently elucidated. Twenty years after the initial diagnosis, we had an opportunity to perform *in situ* hybridization using probes for EBV-encoded small nuclear RNA (EBER) on his paraffin-embedded samples. Numerous EBER (+) cells were found in the skin lesions. Our case previously reported as HV and malignant lymphoma in 1986 was finally diagnosed as EBV-associated NK/T cell lymphoprolifelative disorder.

Fig. 1: Edematous face with induration (a), vesicles, ulcers and crusts on dorsa of hands (b), ulcer and scar on ear lobe (c). Necrotic epidermis and dense cell infiltrate in deep dermis (×10, d). High magnification of Fig. D. Atypical lymphoid cells in deep dermis and fatty tissue (×200, e). Destruction of the original architecture. Infiltration of histiocytic cells and atypical lymphocytes. (×400, Cervical lymph node, f). Autopsy findings. Actinomycosis in lung (g), hemophagocytosis in bone marrow (h) and liver (i). Numerous EBER(+) cells infiltrated in dermis (j) under vesicle (ISH, k).

References

Oono T, Arata J, Masuda T et al. (1986) Coexistence of hydroa vacciniforme and malignant lymphoma. Arch Dermatol 122:1306–1309

Iwatsuki K, Xu Z, Takata M et al. (1999) The association of latent Epstein-Barr virus infection with hydroa vacciniforme. Brt J Dermatol 140:715–721

Iwatsuki K, Ohtsuka K, Harada H et al. (1997) Clinicopathologic manifestations of Epstein-Barr virus-associated cutaneous lymphoproliferative disorders. Arch Dermatol 133:1081–1086

Iwatsuki K, Yamamoto T, Tsuji K et al. (2004) A spectrum of clinical manifestations caused by host immune responses against Epstein-Barr virus infections. Acta Med Okayama 58:169–180

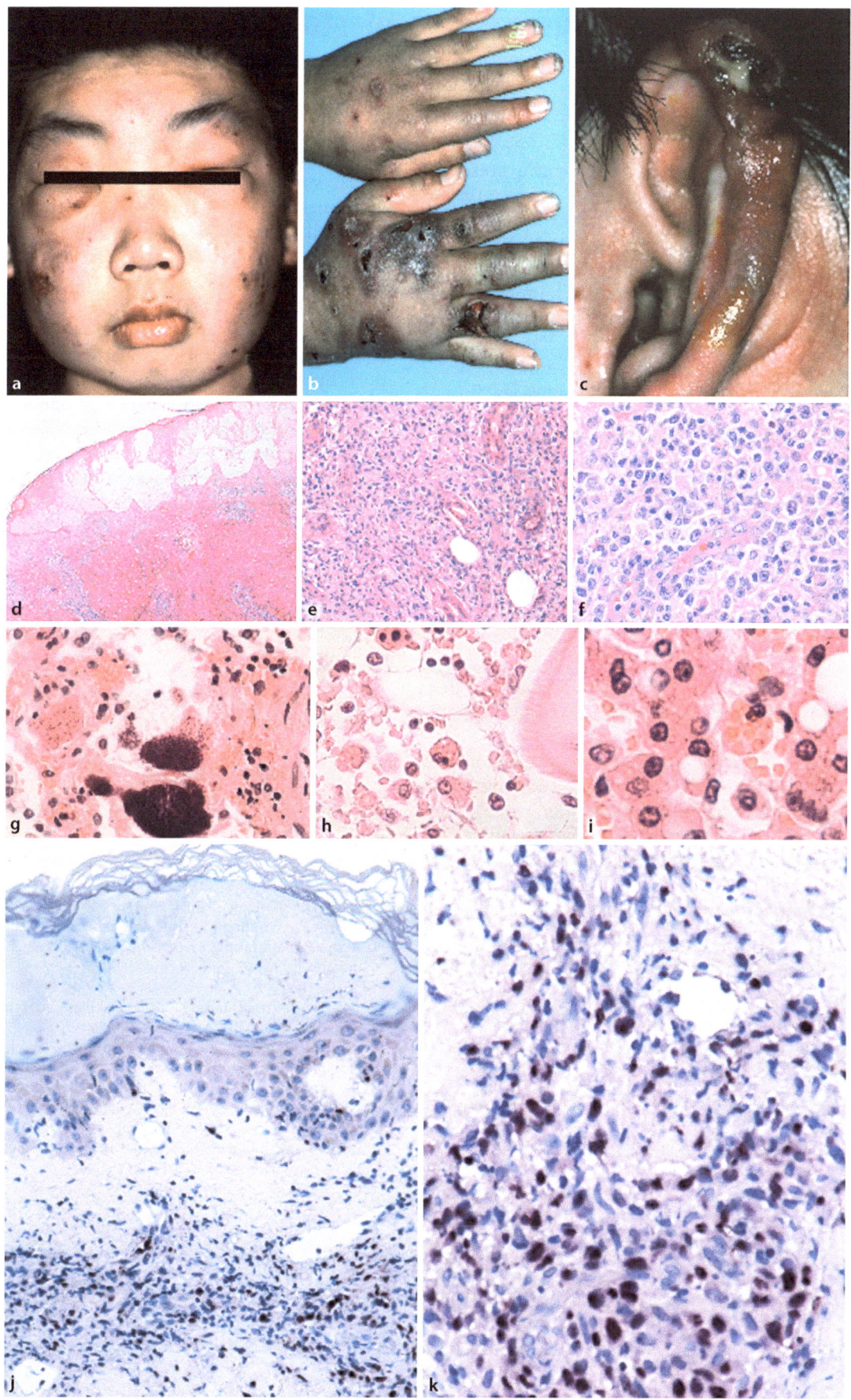

Epstein-Barr virus-positive blastoid NK-cell lymphoma

T. Sale, G. S. Wood and B. J. Longley

Age: 77 years   **Sex:** F

Clinical features: A 77-year-old female presented with rapidly growing violaceous plaques on her scalp, face, trunk, and upper extremities. She had no nasopharyngeal lesions and no palpable lymphadenopathy. Histopathologic examination demonstrated dermal aggregates of large cells with hyperchromatic and angulated nuclei which varied in size and shape. The aggregates followed vascular, neural, and adnexal structures and invaded arrector pili muscles. Tumor cells stained positive for CD56, CD45, CD31, and EBER. Negative staining was seen for CD1a, CD3, CD5, CD20, CD21, CD30, CD34, CD68, CD117, myeloperoxidase, S-100 protein, and TIA-l. Bone marrow analysis was additionally positive for CD38 and negative for CD8 and TdT. CT scan of the chest, abdomen, and pelvis demonstrated mild axillary lymphadenopathy and marked splenomegaly.

Diagnosis: Blastoid NK-cell lymphoma.

Follow-up: Chemotherapy was initiated with pentostatin. Initial improvement was seen with the first dose but growth of tumors resumed after the second dose. Pentostatin was discontinued. Weekly gemcytabine was begun with significant improvement by week three of therapy and resolution of all but one visible skin lesion by the third month of treatment. One month later, the patient missed two doses of gemcytabine due to thrombocytopenia and soon after her disease relapsed.

Comment: Blastoid Natural killer (NK)-cell lymphoma is one of the four subtypes of NK-cell lymphoma recognized by the World Health Organization 2001 classification scheme. Unlike nasal and nasal-type NK/T cell lymphomas, blastoid NK-cell lymphoma generally presents in non-Asian populations. Development of bruise-like or petechial skin lesions occurs along with involvement of bone marrow, lymph nodes, and peripheral blood. Immunostaining is positive for CD56 and CD4 and negative for CD57, surface CD3, and markers of cytotoxic molecules. Histopathology demonstrates medium- and large-sized cells with a blastic morphology, inconspicuous cytoplasmic granules, absence of angiodestruction, and no zonal necrosis. Most cases of blastoid NK-cell lymphoma have been described as Epstein-Barr virus (EBV) negative. Similar to our case, a recent report by Ling et al. describes an Epstein-Barr virus-positive blastoid NK-cell lymphoma in a Caucasian. Prognosis in blastoid NK-cell lymphoma is poor. Reports of therapy with single- and multi-agent chemotherapeutic regimens as well as allogeneic stem cell transplantation have been described.

- **Fig. 1:** Violaceous nodules present on the face.
- **Fig. 2:** Scattered violaceous and petechial lesions on the trunk.
- **Fig. 3:** Dense dermal infiltrate with grenz zone, H & E ×2.
- **Fig. 4:** H & E ×60.
- **Fig. 5:** CD56 staining.
- **Fig. 6:** CD45 staining.
- **Fig. 7:** CD31 staining.

References

Kazakov DV, Mentzel T, Burg G et al. (2003) Blastic natural killer-cell lymphoma of the skin associated with myelodysplastic syndrome or myelogenous leukaemia: a coincidence or more? Br J Dermatol 149:869–876

Ling TC, Harris M, Craven NM (2002) Epstein-Barr virus-positive blastoid nasal T/natural killer-cell lymphoma in a Caucasian. Br J Dermatol 146:700–703

Shapiro M, Wasik MA, Junkins-Hopkins J et al. (2003) Complete remission in advanced blastic NK-cell lymphoma/leukemia in elderly patients using the hyper-CVAD regimen. Am J Hematol 74:46–51

Uchiyama N, Ito K, Kawai K et al. (1998) CD2−, CD4+, CD56+ agranular natural killer cell lymphoma of the skin. Am J Dermpath 20:513–517

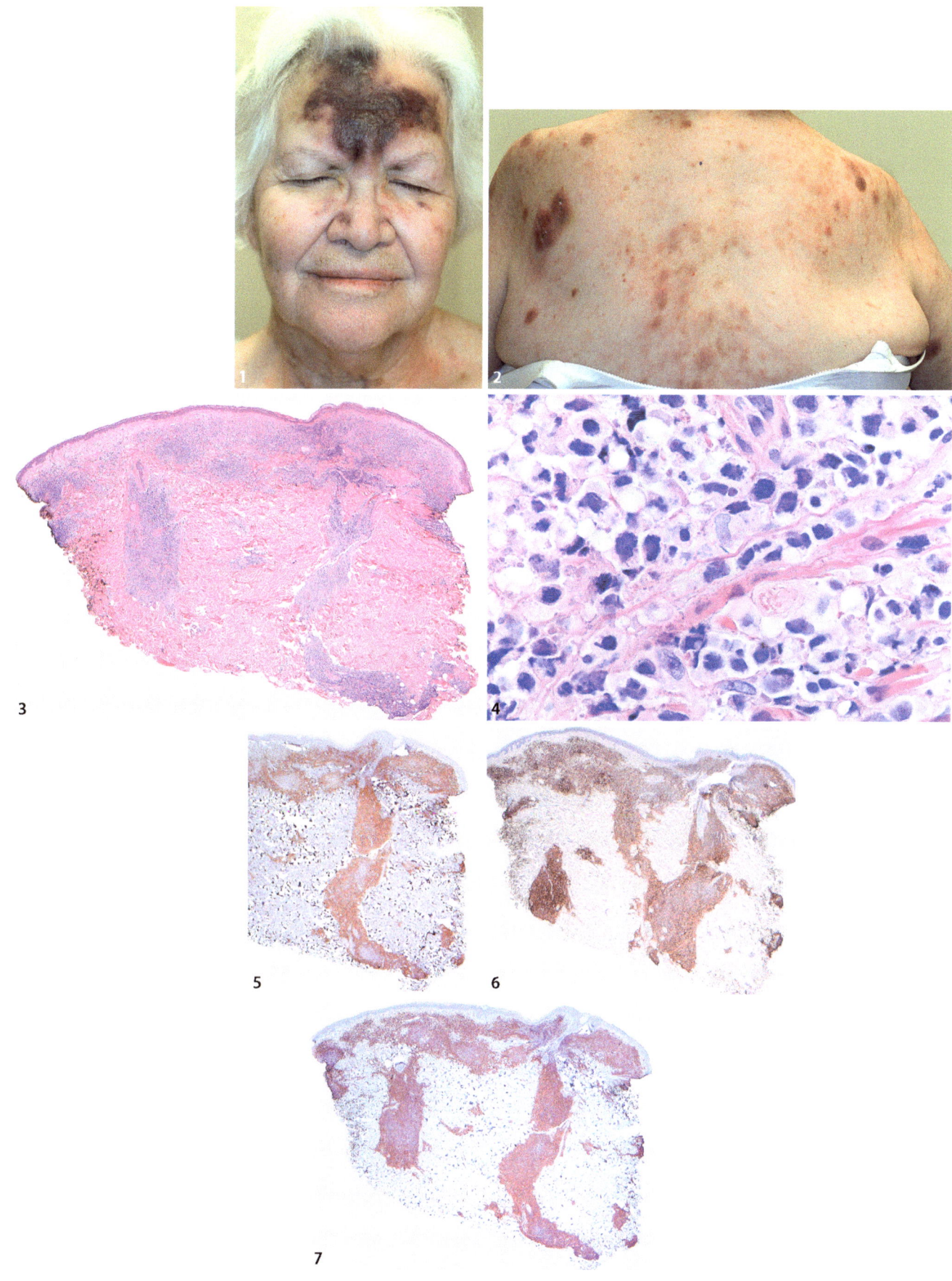

2 Mature B-cell Neoplasms

2.1 Cutaneous Marginal Zone B-cell Lymphoma (MALT Type)

■ Primary cutaneous marginal zone B-cell lymphoma with secondary anetoderma in a patient with Sjögren's syndrome

M. H. Vermeer, J. Hoefnagel, P. M. Jansen, C. J. L. M. Meijer and R. Willemze

Age: 49 years   **Sex:** F

Clinical features: The patient presented with a three-year history of an increasing number of well-circumscribed, firm and erythematous plaques and nodules on the trunk that resolved spontaneously leaving skin-colored to lightly pigmented atrophic areas.

Fourteen years earlier she was diagnosed with Sjögren's syndrome. Histology from an enlarged parotid gland showed a diffuse proliferation of B-cells, but no signs of malignant transformation. *Borrelia* serology was negative and protein electrophoresis was normal.

Diagnosis: Primary cutaneous marginal zone B-cell lymphoma with secondary anetoderma in a patient with Sjögren's syndrome.

Follow-up: Because the patient had no complaints of the skin lesions no therapy was started. During follow up a small number of new erythematous nodules appeared, some of which have resolved spontaneously leaving clinical anetoderma. The swelling in the parotid gland resolved spontaneously.

Comment: Anetoderma is a circumscribed area of slack skin with loss of dermal substance on palpation due to a localized loss in elastic tissue. Primary anetoderma is defined as cases where no underlying associated disease can be identified. Secondary anetoderma is seen in inflammatory cutaneous diseases including discoid and systemic lupus erythematosus, antiphospholipid syndrome, acne, Wells syndrome and cutaneous infections such as herpes zoster, borreliosis, human immunodeficiency virus and syphilis. Skin neoplasms including pilomatricoma and B-cell lymphomas are less common causes of anetoderma.

This patient illustrates the association of cutaneous B-cell lymphoproliferative disease and anetoderma. One previous report regarded a 64-year-old man with Sjögren's syndrome who developed anetodermic lesions associated with a cutaneous plasmacytoma and a 32-year old man with anetodermic lesions associated with B-cell cutaneous hyperplasia. In two recent reports a total of four patients were presented with anetoderma associated with immunocytoma (two patients), marginal zone B-cell lymphoma (one patient) and post-transplant B-cell lymphoproliferative disorder (one patient).

Anetoderma without detectable, underlying skin disease has been described in two patients with Sjögren's which may illustrate that patients with Sjögren's disease have an increased propensity for elastic tissue loss.

▥ **Fig. 1:** An erythematous nodule on the abdomen.

▥ **Fig. 2:** Flaccid hanging nodule on the back after resolution of erythematous nodule.

▥ **Fig. 3:** Secondary anetoderma on the abdomen after resolution of erythematous nodule.

▥ **Fig. 4:** Heavy lymphoid infiltrate extending to the deep reticular dermis.

▥ **Fig. 5:** Perivascular infiltrate containing lymphocytes and plasma cells in the papillary dermis.

▥ **Fig. 6:** Plasmacytoid cells stained strongly for kappa but not for lambda.

▥ **Fig. 7:** Elastin Verhoeff-van Gieson's stain demonstrates loss and fragmentation of dermal elastic tissue fibers.

References

Jubert C, Cosnes A, Wechsler J, Andre P, Revuz J, Bagot M (1995) Anetoderma may reveal cutaneous plasmacytoma and benign cutaneous lymphoid hyperplasia. Arch Dermatol 131:365–366

Kasper RC, Wood GS, Nihal M, LeBoit PE (2001) Anetoderma arising in cutaneous B-cell lymphoproliferative disease. Am J Dermatopathol 23:124–132

Child FJ, Woollons A, Price ML, Calonje E, Russell-Jones R (2000) Multiple cutaneous immunocytoma with secondary anetoderma: a report of two cases. Br J Dermatol 143:165–170

Torne R, Su WPD, Winkelmann RK, Smolle J, Kerl H (1990) Clinicopathologic study of cutaneous plasmacytoma. Int J Dermatol 29:562–566

Herrero-Gonzalez JE, Herrero-Mateu C (2002) Primary anetoderma associated with primary Sjogren's syndrome. Lupus 11:124–126

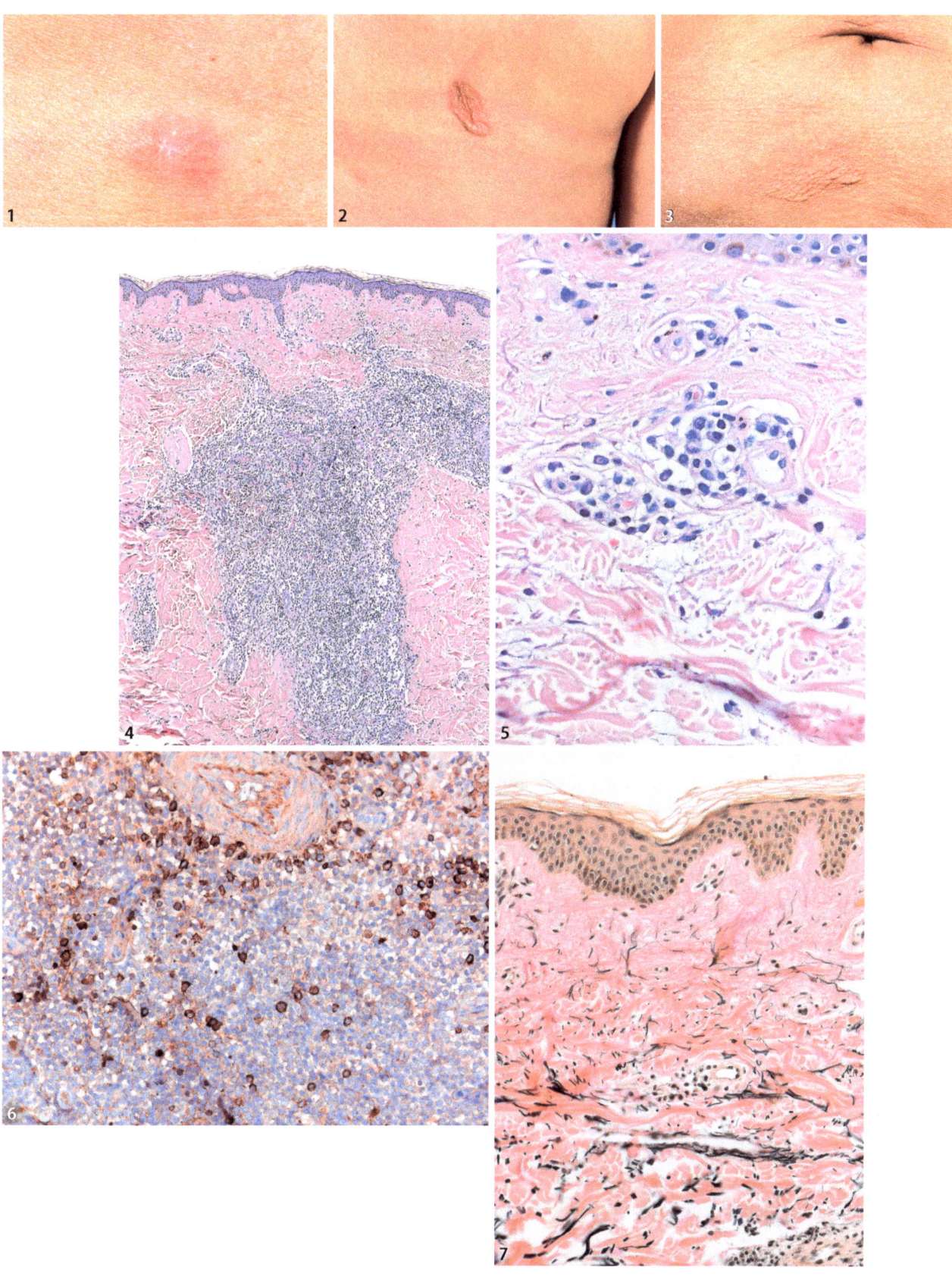

Follicular lymphoma with follicular dendritic cell overgrowth

D. V. KAZAKOV, L. BOUDOVA and M. MICHAL

Age: 87 years   **Sex:** F

Clinical features: The patient presented with an asymptomatic, subcutaneous nodule 2.5 cm in diameter located on her breast. The lesion was surgically excised. Clinical investigation revealed diffuse signet ring-cell carcinoma of the stomach and adenocarcinoma of the colon. No extracutaneous lymphoma was found.

Diagnosis: Follicular lymphoma of the skin and subcutis with a prominent follicular dendritic cell proliferation.

Follow-up: The patient was considered inoperable and died 8 months later. No autopsy was performed.

Comment: The most striking feature of the lesion is the extensive proliferation of follicular dendritic cells (FDC) which masked the lymphoma by obscuring a typical follicular growth pattern. In follicular lymphoma, meshworks of FDC are constantly present in the neoplastic follicles and may also be noted outside them as small, delicate islands. Cases of follicular lymphoma in which FDC outnumber lymphoma cells are extremely rare. FDC are mainly considered to be reactive in follicular lymphoma, although the possibility that they represent a part of the neoplastic clone has been entertained. The indirect proof of the reactive nature of the FDC proliferation in our case is the sharp circumscription of the lesion. Such a prominent FDC overgrowth may be due to costimulatory interactions between FDC and germinal center cells. Main differential diagnoses included FDC tumor/sarcoma and the "stroma-rich" variant of the hyaline-vascular type of Castleman disease.

- **Fig. 1:** A striking pallor of the lesion that is predominantly composed of follicular dendritic cells arranged in fascicles, whorls, and round islands.
- **Fig. 2:** Follicular dendritic cells with large elongated or oval pale nuclei with fine chromatin, small distinct nucleoli and a delicate nuclear membrane. The cytoplasm is ample and pale to faintly eosinophilic, with indistinct cellular borders.
- **Fig. 3:** Follicular dendritic cells are intimately intermingled with centroblasts and centrocytes, some of which are slightly pleomorphic (Giemsa staining). This close association of the lymphoma cells with follicular dendritic cells was seen throughout the whole lesion. Nowhere in the lesion was there an independently growing lymphoma or a follicular dendritic cell tumor. Neither follicular dendritic cells nor lymphoma cells sprinkled over the sharp margin of the tumoral mass.
- **Fig. 4:** A follicular growth pattern was mainly seen at the periphery of the lesion.
- **Fig. 5:** A close-up view of the lymphoid follicle depicted in Fig. 4: note the predominance of follicular dendritic cells in the germinal center and a reduced mantle zone.
- **Fig. 6:** Follicular dendritic cells are stained with CD35. Germinal center cells were immunoreactive for CD10, CD20, CD79a, and bcl-6 (not shown).

References

Kazakov DV, Palmedo G, Mukensnabl P et al. (2004) Follicular lymphoma of the skin and superficial soft tissues associated with a prominent follicular dendritic cell proliferation: an unusual pattern which may represent a diagnostic pitfall. Pathol Res Pract 200:557–565

Chan JCK (1997) Proliferative lesions of follicular dendritic cells: an overview, including a detailed account of follicular dendritic cells sarcoma, a neoplasm with many faces and uncommon etiologic associations. Adv Anat Pathol 4:357–411

Liu YJ, Grouard G, de Bouteiller O et al. (1996) Follicular dendritic cells and germinal centers. Int Rev Cytol 166:139–179

Kazakov DV, Fanburg-Smith JC, Suster S et al. (2004) Castleman disease of the subcutis and underlying skeletal muscle: report of 6 cases. Am J Surg Pathol 28:569–577

Danon AD, Krishnan J, Frizzera G (1993) Morpho-immunophenotypic diversity of Castleman's disease, hyaline-vascular type: with emphasis on a stroma-rich variant and a new pathogenetic hypothesis. Virchows Arch A Pathol Anat Histopathol 423:369–382

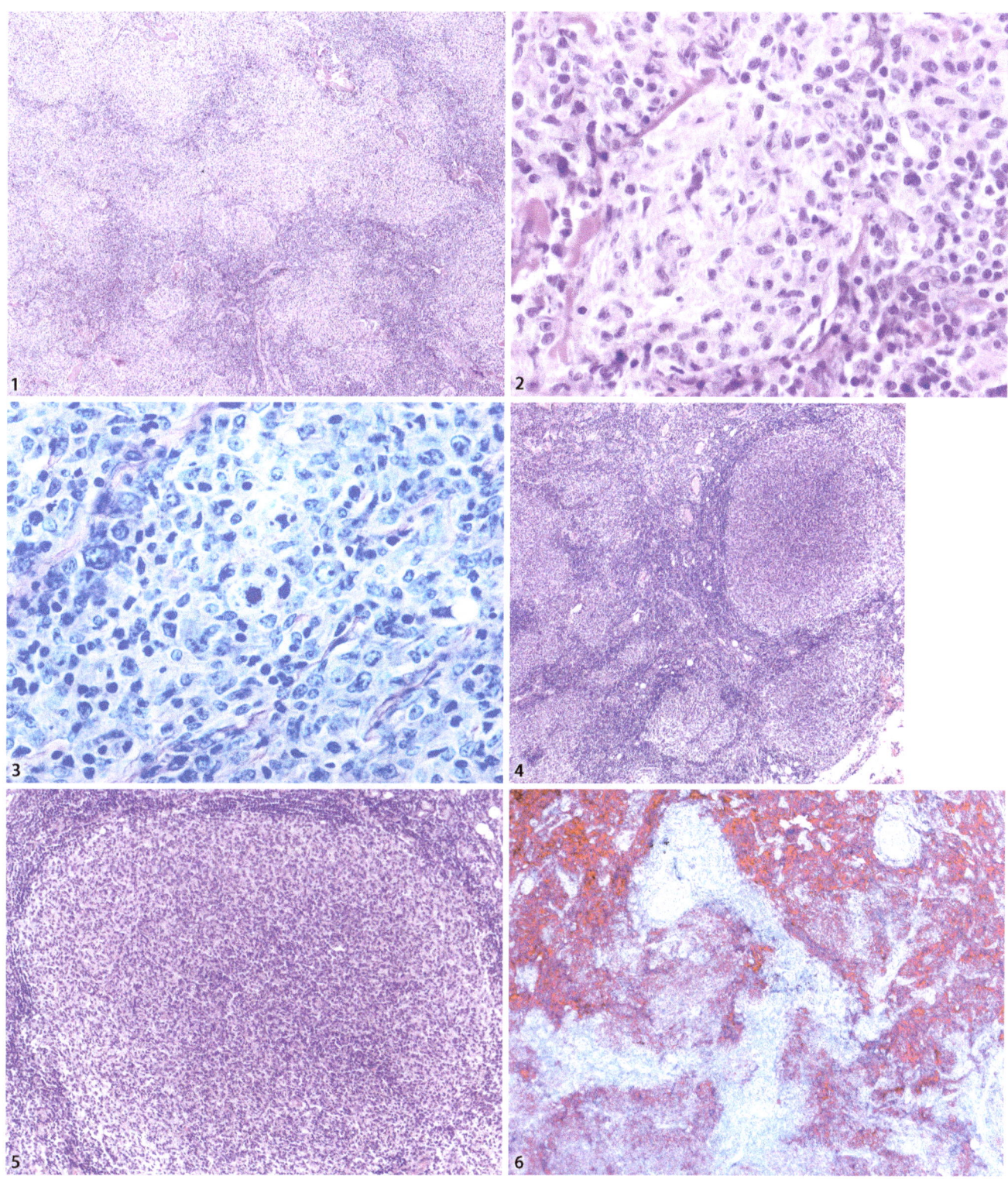

Diffuse large B-cell lymphoma with cutaneous and ocular involvement

W. Kempf, Ph. Golling, B. Christen, M. Messmer, S. Michaelis, G. Burg and R. Dummer

Age: 67 years   **Sex:** F

Clinical features: The patient suffered since 1 year from a slowly enlarging, gyrated and erythematous infiltration on the left arm. No B-symptoms, no hepatosplenomegaly or lymphadenopathy were present and bone marrow biopsy showed normal findings. Staging did not reveal extracutaneous involvement except for pseudophakia and infiltration of the vitreal body of both eyes. MRI did not reveal any involvement of central nervous system by lymphoma. Vitrectomy on the right eye and cytologic analysis demonstrated infiltration by atypical lymphoid cells similar to the tumor cells found in the skin biopsy. Genotyping of cutaneous lymphoma by Southern blot analysis was not conclusive for rearrangement of Ig heavy chain genes. The t(14;18) translocation was not found and serology for Borrelia was negative.

Diagnosis: Diffuse large B-cell lymphoma with cutaneous and ocular involvement.

Follow-up: Radiotherapy (2200 cGy) led to complete regression of the cutaneous tumor. The ocular involvement was not treated, since the patient did not experience visual impairment. Two months after radiotherapy, local recurrence of cutaneous lymphoma was observed. Systemic interferon alpha 2 a (3 Mio IU three times weekly subcutaneously) and radiotherapy (up to 4600 cGy) was initiated.

Comment: Cutaneous diffuse large B-cell lymphoma (DLBCL) occurs mostly on the legs of elderly women and shows histologically diffuse, cohesive infiltrates of large B-cells with round nuclei and prominent nucleoli resembling centroblasts and immunoblasts. In our patient, the tumor was located on the left arm and histologically composed of large B-cells scattered or arranged in small clusters in a background infiltrate of numerous small CD3+ T-cells. The tumor cells expressed bcl-6 and bcl-2. Based on these features, this lymphoma belongs to the group of "DLBCL, others" according to the

WHO/EORTC classification. In regard to the histologic pattern, the lesion has features of a cutaneous T-cell rich B-cell lymphoma. Simultaneous involvement of the skin and ocular structures have not been reported so far in DLBCL. The ocular involvement raises the question whether this tumor represents in fact a primary cutaneous B-cell lymphoma with ocular involvement or an ocular lymphoma with cutaneous involvement.

- **Fig. 1:** Gyrated and erythematous infiltrated skin lesions on the left arm.
- **Fig. 2:** Dense confluent lymphocytic infiltration of the entire dermis. HE, microscopic magnification 25×.
- **Fig. 3:** Large lymphoid tumor cells are present scattered or arranged in small clusters, embedded in a background of numerous small lymphocytes (**a**) and detail (**b**).
- **Fig. 4:** The large tumor cells express CD20 and represent centroblast and immunoblast-like B-cells.
- **Fig. 5:** Expression of bcl-2 by the tumor cells.
- **Fig. 6:** Tumor cells from ocular involvement (cytologic preparation of vitrectomy specimen).

References

Burg G et al (2005) Cutaneous diffuse large B-cell lymphoma. In: LeBoit P, Weedon D, Burg G, Vardiman JW (eds) WHO Classification of Skin Tumors. Pathology and Genetics. IARC Press, Lyon

Coupland SE, Bechrakis NE, Anastassiou G et al. (2003) Evaluation of vitrectomy specimens and chorioretinal biopsies in the diagnosis of primary intraocular lymphoma in patients with Masquerade syndrome. Graefes Arch Clin Exp Ophthalmol 241:860–870

Goodlad JR, Krajewski AS, Batstone PJ et al. (2003) Primary cutaneous diffuse large B-cell lymphoma. Prognostic significance and clinicopathologic subtypes. Am J Surg Pathol 27:1538–1545

Grange F, Bekkenk MW, Wechsler J et al. (2001) Prognostic factors in primary cutaneous large B-cell lymphomas: A European multicenter study. J Clin Oncol 19:3602–3610

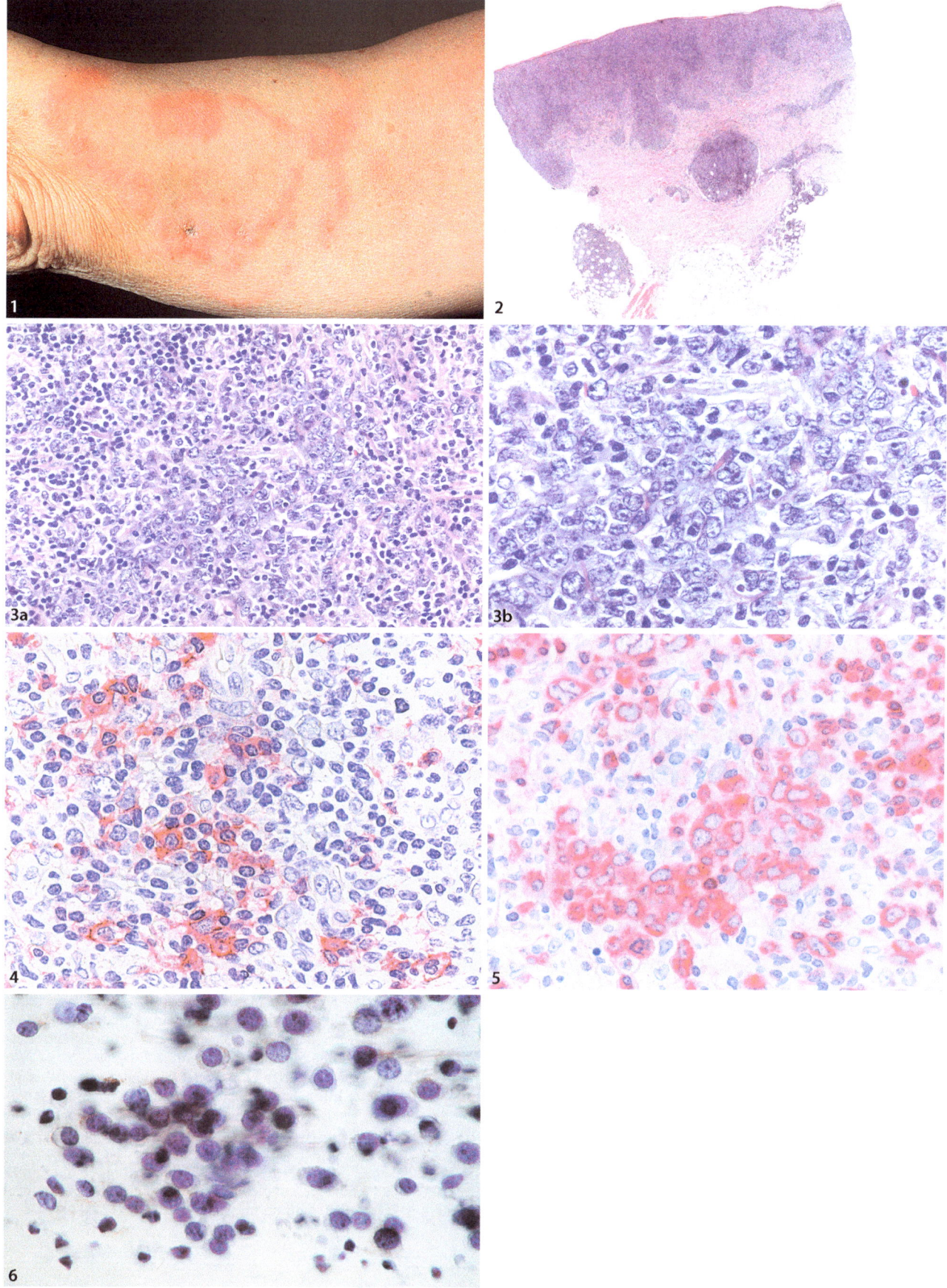

EBV-positive cutaneous B-cell lymphoproliferative disease after imatinib mesylate (Glivec)

M. W. Bekkenk, M. H. Vermeer, C. J. L. M. Meijer, P. M. Jansen, J. M. Middeldorp, S. J. C. Stevens and R. Willemze

Age: 70 years   **Sex:** F

Clinical features: This patient was reffered from the hematology department, where she was known with a chronic myeloid leukemia (CML). She was previously treated with 1000 mg hydroxyurea twice daily, resulting in stable disease. However, upon development of a leg ulcer, hydroxyurea was discontinued and ambulant compression therapy in combination with 2×200 mg/d pentoxyfilline (PTX) and 100 mg/d ascal was initiated. Her CML progressed, and 500 mg/d imatinib mesylate was started. Subsequently, her leukocyte count decreased from 9.9×10^9/L before treatment to 1.3×10^9/L after 2 months of treatment. Shortly after starting imatinib mesylate she noticed a rapidly growing, ulcerating tumor on her head. A biopsy showed a diffuse proliferation of large, atypical, immunoblastic B cells that strongly expressed CD79a and CD30 and were monotypic immunoglobulin G (IgG) lambda-positive. Most large atypical cells stained positive for EBV-encoded RNA1 (EBER-1), mRNAs, and latent membrane protein 1 (LMP-1) and EBV nuclear antigen 1 (EBNA1) proteins, whereas focal expression was found for BamHI fragment Z left frame 1 (BZLF1). There was no expression for EBV early antigen (EA), EBV viral capsid antigen (VCA), and membrane antigen (MA). RNA in situ hybridization showed expression of EBER-1 and EBER-2. An immunoblot assay and synthetic peptide ELISA test demonstrated a strong IgG response against VCA (p18 – p40) and the lytic switch protein Zebra. There was a high IgA response against VCA (P18), without significant reactivity to other EBV antigens. Combined, these findings are consistent with EBV-related lymphoproliferation due to EBV reactivation and persistent EBV replication. Staging procedures were negative.

Diagnosis: EBV-positive cutaneous B-cell lymphoproliterative disease after imatinib mesylate (Glivec).

Follow-up: The dose of the imatinib mesylate was lowered to 400 mg/d. This resulted in a rise in the patient's leukocyte count to 2.8×10^9/L and spontaneous resolution of the tumor.

Comment: EBV-associated lymphoid proliferations are a heterogeneous group of lymphoproliferative diseases occurring in the setting of immunosuppression in which the level of T-cell depletion is considered to be one of the most important risk factors. Primary cutaneous EBV-associated B-cell lymphoproliferative disease generally has a good prognosis, and after recovery of the immunocompromised status a spontaneous remission often is observed. The spontaneous remission of the tumor after restoration of the leukocyte count in the presented patient is in line with these observations. Early recognition of EBV-related posttransplantation lymphoproliferative disease is crucial, because in these early phases restoration of immunosuppression may still result in disappearance of the lesions. In later stages, when a frank lymphoma develops, treatment is more difficult and the prognosis is not as good.

- **Fig. 1:** Ulcerating tumor on the scalp (**a**) and spontaneous resolution after lowering dosage of imatinib mesylate (**b**).
- **Fig. 2:** Diffuse proliferation of large atypical blasts.

References

Gross TG, Steinbuch M, DeFor T et al. (1999) B cell lymphoproliferative disorders following hematopoietic stem cell transplantation: risk factors, treatment and outcome. Bone Marrow Transplant 23:251–258

Blokx WAM, Andriessen MPM, van Hamersvelt HW et al. (2002) Initial spontaneous remission of posttransplantation Epstein Barr Virus-related B-cell lymphoproliferative disorder of the skin in a renal transplant recipient. Am J Dermatopathol 24:414–422

Bekkenk MW, Vermeer MH, Meijer CJLM et al. (2003) EBV-positive cutaneous B-cell lymphoproliferative disease after imatinib mesylate. Blood 102:4243–4244

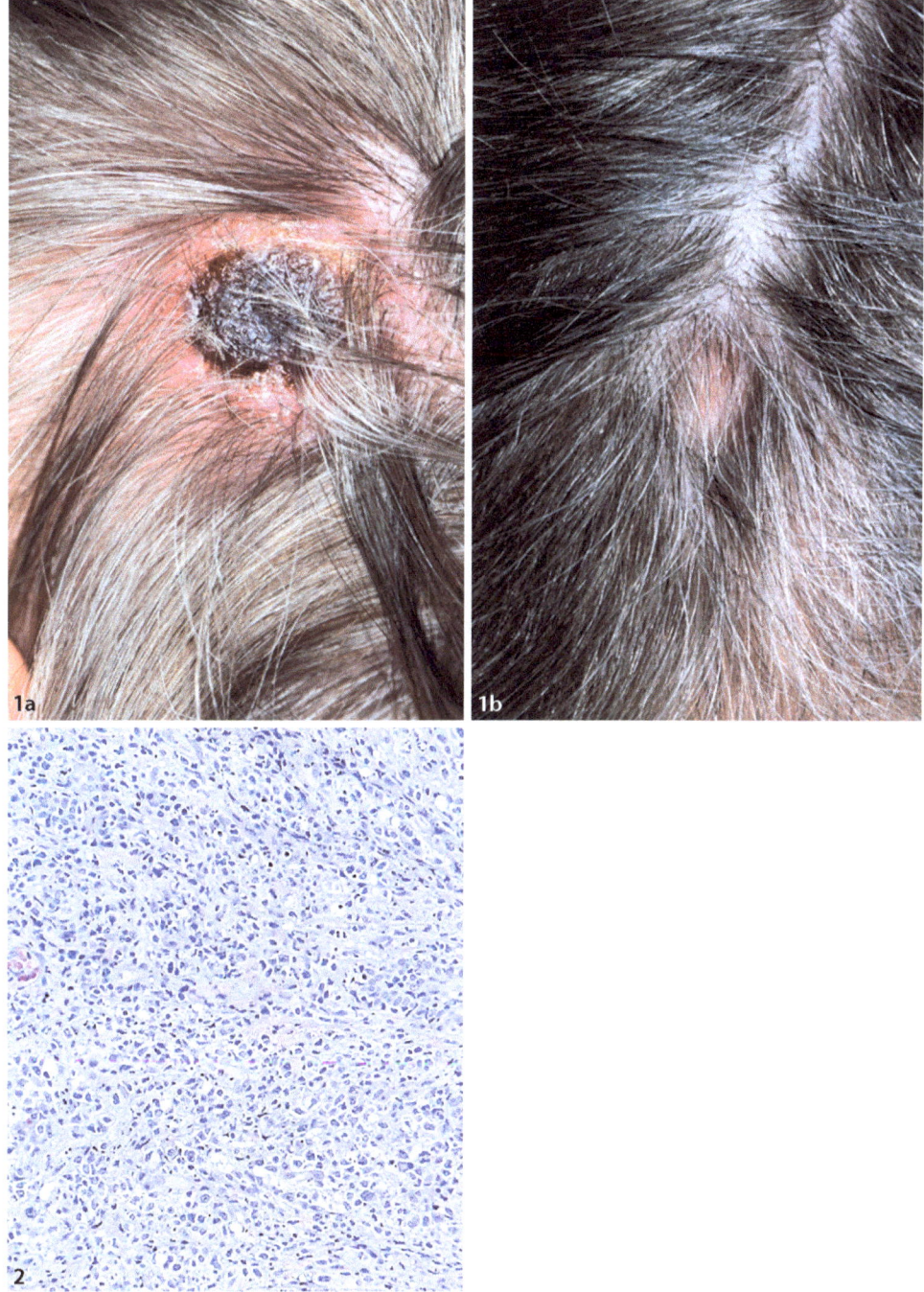

B-cell chronic lymphocytic leukemia revealed by an erythroderma

G. Quereux and B. Dreno

Age: 70 years   **Sex:** M

Clinical features: Polymorphic papular rash with annular lesions on the trunk and erythematous patches on the legs appeared 6 months earlier. Secondarily, during the course of a few days we observed spontaneous decrease of these lesions followed by the appearance of a dry and pruriginous erythroderma. It was associated with hyperkeratosis of the palms and soles, bilateral ectropion and lymphadenopathy in the axillae and groin, simulating Sézary syndroma.

The histology found a sparse dermal infiltrate of lymphocytes. Most of those were CD2+, CD3+, CD4+ T cell, and only a few lymphocytes were CD 20+.

The white blood cell count showed an hyperlymphocytosis ($7000/cm^3$). Immunochemistry demonstrated the presence of 45% of typical lymphocytic leukaemia (CLL) B cells and 55% of atypical cells mimicking Sézary cells CD26–.

CLL involved bone marrow and peripheric lymph node.

No clonality was found using T-cell receptor gene analysis both in the circulating lymphocytes, the skin and the lymph node.

CT scan (thoracic and abdominal) and abdominal ultrasonography were negative.

Diagnosis: B cell chronic lymphocytic leukemia revealed by an erythroderma.

Follow-up: Five months of PUVA therapy resulted only in a partial remission. Phototherapy was therefore discontinued and systemic retinoid (acitretin) started. Three months later we noted a complete disappearance of the erythroderma.

Comment: Cutaneous lesions arising during the course of CLL are frequent, but the specific lesions represent only 10% of the cases. Those are very polymorphic: tumours, nodules, scaly erythematous patches, infiltrated violaceous papules on the face (especially on the nose and the ears), and erythroderma (4.5%). The histology of these lesions is characterized by the presence of an infiltrate consisting primarily of small lymphocytes located in the perivascular and periadnexal regions.

This observation is original for two reasons. First, the patient really looks like a Sézary syndrome with palmoplantar hyperkeratosis. On the biological level, it's surprising to find two different subpopulations of lymphocytes with 45% of cells of B cell CLL CD38+ and in addition 55% of CD26– cells mimicking Sézary cells. This raises the assumption of an inductive role of the T-"Sézary"-cells in the development of the population of B cell lymphocytes, by notably secretion of cytokines.

Fig. 1: Erythematous and annular papules on the axillae.
Fig. 2: Erythematous and annular papules on the abdomen.
Fig. 3: Erythroderma.
Fig. 4: Erythroderma.
Fig. 5: Palmar hyperkeratosis.

References

Bonvalet D, Foldes C, Civatte J (1984) Cutaneous manifestations in chronic lymphocytic leukemia. J Dermatol Surg Oncol 10:278–282

Cerroni L, Zenahlik P, Hofler G, Kaddu S, Kerl H (1996) Specific cutaneous infiltrates of B-cell chronic lymphocytic leukemia: has clinicopathologic and prognostic study of 42 patients. Am J Surg Pathol 20:1000–1010

Volk AI, Vannuci SA, Cook W, Thompson KA, Listinsky CM (2002) Composite mycosis fungoides and B-cell chronic lymphocytic leukemia. Ann Diagn Pathol 6:172–182

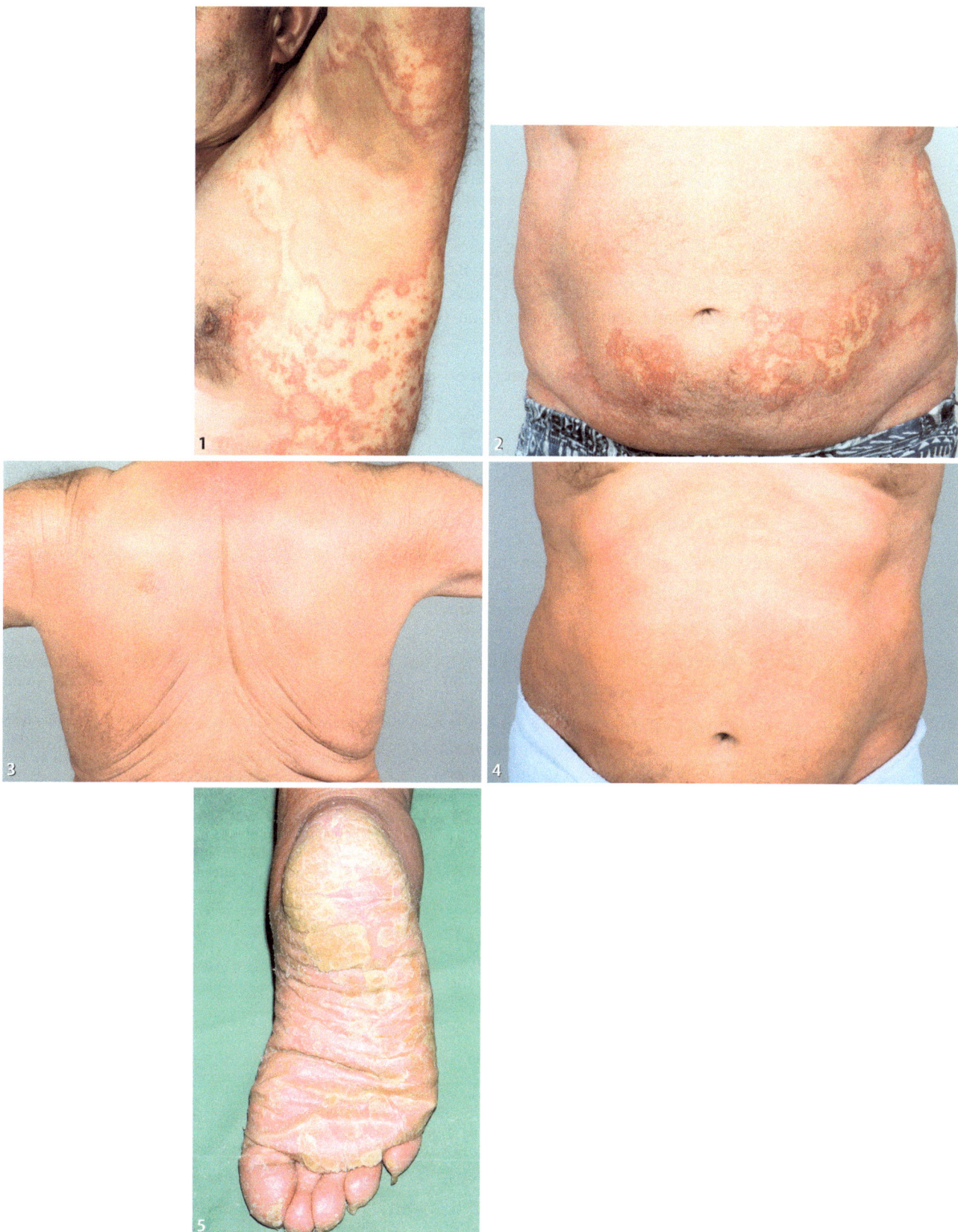

B-cell chronic lymphocytic leukemia (B-CLL) at the site of Borrelia burgdorferi infection

L. Cerroni and H. Kerl

Age: 58 years   **Sex:** F

Clinical features: Solitary nodule on the left nipple for the last few weeks. The clinical presentation was suggestive of Borrelia burgdorferi-associated lymphocytoma cutis. The patient had B-cell chronic lymphocytic leukemia (B-CLL) managed without specific treatment at the time of onset of skin lesions.

Diagnosis: Borrelia burgdorferi-associated specific cutaneous infiltrate of B-CLL.

Follow-up: Molecular analyses revealed the presence of specific DNA sequences of Borrelia burgdorferi, indicating that the skin lesions were triggered by a Borrelia infection.

Comment: Specific skin infiltrates of B-CLL at sites of cutaneous inflammation, including among others infections due to herpes virus or inflammatory infiltrates surrounding skin tumors, are well known. Onset of specific lesions at sites typical for Borrelia burgdorferi-induced lymphocytoma cutis (nipple, earlobe, scrotum), too, is not uncommon in these patients. Especially the presence of leukemic infiltrates on the nipple is described in old textbooks as "leukemia lymphatica mamillae", and was considered in the past as a typical specific cutaneous presentation of B-CLL. We demonstrated that these particular cases represent in fact specific manifestations of B-CLL induced by infection with Borrelia burgdorferi. Histopathologic features in Borrelia-associated skin infiltrates in B-CLL patients are characterized by dense perivascular and periadnexal infiltrates of small hyperchromatic lymphocytes throughout the entire dermis reaching the subcutaneous fat. Immunohistology reveals an aberrant CD20+/CD5+ phenotype of neoplastic B cells. Molecular analyses show a monoclonal pattern of J_H gene rearrangement, and presence of Borrelia-specific DNA sequences. Skin manifestations of B-CLL induced by Borrelia infection may respond to antibiotic treatment.

- **Fig. 1:** Solitary erythematous nodule on the nipple. The clinical features are identical to those of so-called Borrelia-lymphocytoma.
- **Fig. 2:** Dense, monomorphous infiltrate throughout the entire specimen. Note absence of germinal centers.
- **Fig. 3:** Small hyperchromatic lymphocytes predominate.
- **Fig. 4:** Immunophenotypic features: positivity for CD20 (**a**) and positivity for CD5 (**b**).

References

Cerroni L, Zenahlik P, Kerl H (1995) Specific cutaneous infiltrates of B-cell chronic lymphocytic leukemia arising at the site of herpes zoster and herpes simplex scars. Cancer 76:26–31

Cerroni L, Zenahlik P, Höfler G et al. (1996) Specific cutaneous infiltrates of B-cell chronic lymphocytic leukemia. A clinicopathologic and prognostic study of 42 patients. Am J Surg Pathol 20:1000–1010

Cerroni L, Höfler G, Bäck B et al. (2002) Specific cutaneous infiltrates of B-cell chronic lymphocytic leukemia (B-CLL) at sites typical for Borrelia burgdorferi infection. J Cut Pathol 29:142–147

Colli C, Leinweber B, Müllegger R et al. (2004) Borrelia burgdorferi-associated lymphocytoma cutis: clinicopathologic, immunophenotypic, and molecular study of 106 cases. J Cut Pathol 31:232–240

Smoller BR, Warnke RA (1998) Cutaneous infiltrate of chronic lymphocytic leukemia and relationship to primary cutaneous epithelial neoplasms. J Cut Pathol 25:160–164

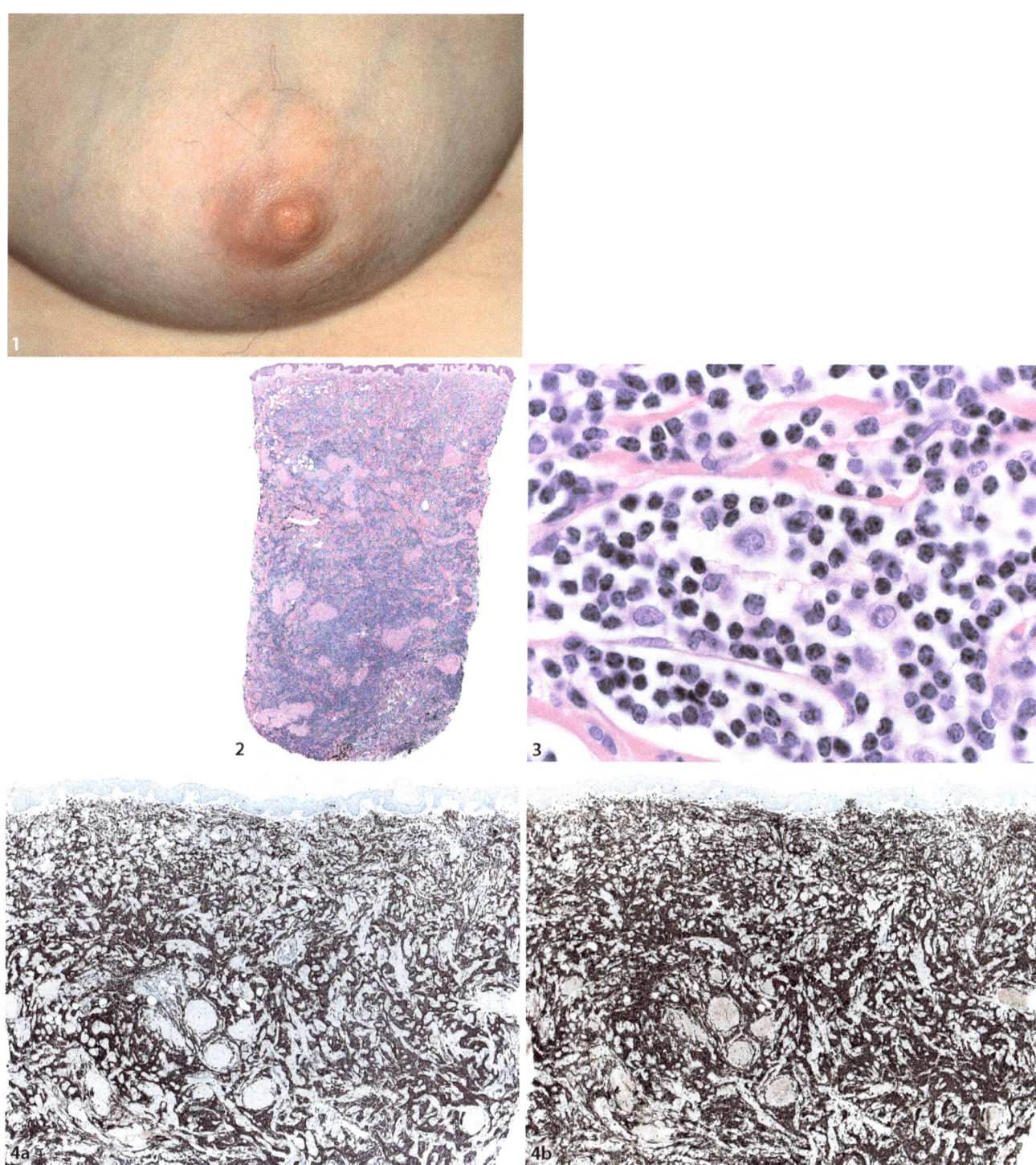

Scarring leukemia cutis

I. E. BELOUSOVA and D. V. KAZAKOV

Age: 79 years   **Sex:** M

Clinical features: One month history of asymptomatic generalized erythematous patches and plaques varying in size and shape. There was moderate bilateral enlargement of the inguinal lymph nodes. Otherwise, the patient was in good general health. A skin biopsy revealed histopathological changes indicative of a lymphoproliferative disorder as well as features of vasculitis. In addition, histologically proven keratoacanthoma was found. Clinical investigation revealed involvement of the bone marrow, peripheral blood (lymphocytosis), peripheral lymph nodes, intra-abdominal lymph nodes, and right suprarenal gland. Histopathological examination of the skin, inguinal lymph nodes, and bone marrow revealed infiltrates of small lymphocytes with scant cytoplasm and clumped chromatin with the following immunophenotype: CD45RB+, CD20+, CD79a+, CD5+, CD23+, CD3−, CD45RO−, cyclin D1−. IgH genes were monoclonally rearranged in the skin and lymph node samples (DNA from bone marrow was not amplifiable).

Diagnosis: B-cell chronic lymphocytic leukemia (B-CLL) with specific cutaneous involvement.

Follow-up: Initially, the patient was only followed-up on inasmuch as he did not fulfill the criteria for starting specific treatment of B-CLL. Five months after the initial presentation, the skin lesions underwent partial spontaneous regression, leaving behind scars on both arms. During the next 1.5 years, the patient experienced several recurrences of skin lesions and their partial spontaneous regression. The scars persisted and remained unchanged. Later, the patient received 3 courses of chemotherapy. At one point, hemorrhagic vesicles appeared around and within the scars, which healed with hyperpigmentation. At his admission, 4.5 years after the initial presentation, the patient was alive and well. Except for the scars, the skin was unremarkable.

Comment: Spontaneous remission of specific skin lesions in B-CLL is rare. When it occurs, it usually has a temporary and partial character. On rare occasions, lesions can fully disappear within days or even several hours leaving normal-appearing skin. Repetitive spontaneous regressions of skin lesions leaving scars are unusual. Vasculitis and edema have been suggested to lead to dermal tissue ischemia and subsequent development of fibrosis/sclerosis.

- **Fig. 1:** Multiple erythematous patches and plaques varying in size and shape.
- **Fig. 2 and 3:** Jagged scars and hyperpigmentation on the patient's arms. The scars appeared at the sites of preexisting, spontaneously resolved lesions. The patient denied any preceding injury to these areas.
- **Fig. 4:** Perivascular lymphoid infiltrates in the upper and mid dermis.
- **Fig. 5:** Small monomorphous lymphoid cells with scant cytoplasm and clumped chromatin.
- **Fig. 6:** Infiltrate within a wall of a medium-sized vessel.

References

Cerroni L, Zenahlik P, Hofler G et al. (1996) Specific cutaneous infiltrates of B-cell chronic lymphocytic leukemia: a clinicopathologic and prognostic study of 42 patients. Am J Surg Pathol 20:1000–1110

Kazakov DV, Belousova IE, Michaelis S et al. (2003) Unusual manifestation of specific cutaneous involvement by B-cell chronic lymphocytic leukemia: spontaneous regression with scar formation. Dermatology 207:111–115

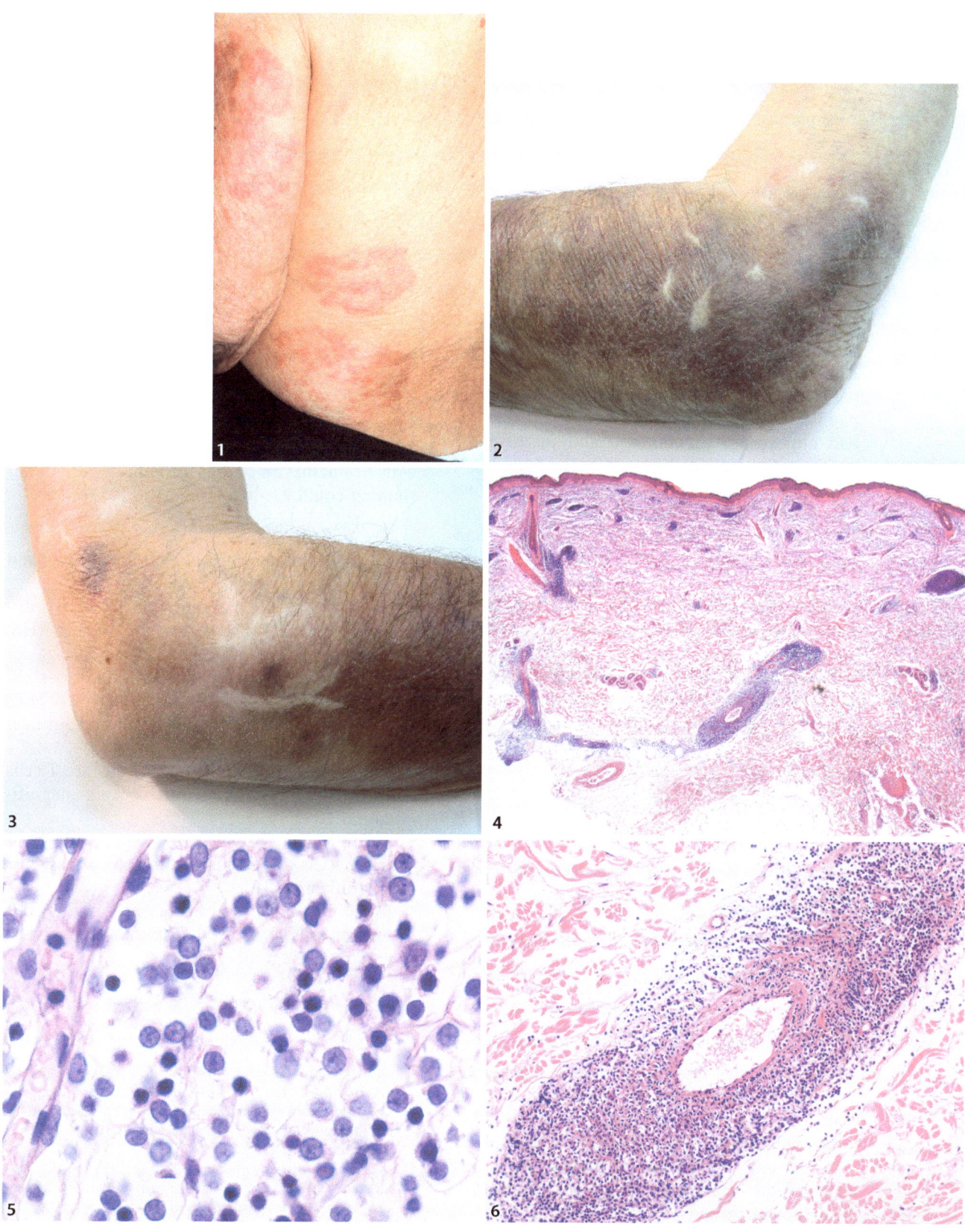

Lymphoma-associated insect bite-like reaction arising in a patient with mantle cell lymphoma

K. Asagoe

Age: 69 years   **Sex:** M

Clinical features: The patient developed systemic lymphadenopathy, and a biopsy from the enlarged lymph node revealed proliferation of medium-sized atypical lymphoid cells that were stained with CD79a+, CD5+, cyclin D1+. He was diagnosed as having mantle cell lymphoma. After his admission, he was referred to our department for evaluation of itchy erythematous papules and nodules on the face and trunk that had appeared 7 months ago and increased in number. The patient had not noticed a history of arthropod assault. Scattered erythematous papules and nodules less than 10 mm in diameter were observed on the face and trunk. Surface lymphadenopathy was marked. A biopsy specimen from the erythematous nodule showed dense nodular lymphocytic infiltration intermingled with eosinophils in the superficial and mid dermis. Immunohistochemical examination revealed that most of the infiltrating cells were T cells and did not express markers suggestive of mantle cell lymphoma, such as cyclin D1.

Diagnosis: Insect bite-like reaction developed in a patient with mantle cell lymphoma.

Follow-up: Although each lesion disappeared within 10 days, new papules developed repeatedly. Topical potent steroidal ointment or oral antihistaminic agents did not work successfully. When the patient received chemotherapy with a large amount of steroid, the lesions disappeared transiently. However, new papules appeared several days after systemic administration of corticosteroid had stopped.

Comment: It has been known that exaggerated reaction to arthropod bite occurs in patients with chronic lymphocytic leukaemia (Davis MD, et al. 1998). Rarely, eruptions similar to arthropod bite reaction develop in patients with hematologic malignant neoplasms without a history of arthropod assaults (Barzilai A, et al. 1999). Although the mechanism of the disease was not well known, altered immune response triggered by neoplastic cells may cause the dis-

ease. Insect bite-like reaction is refractory to the treatment and only a large amount of systemic corticosteroid is known to be effective.

On the other hand, skin involvement of mantle cell lymphoma, which manifests as nodules, macules, maculopapular rush and plaques, very rarely occurs (Sen F, et al. 2002). Histologically, perivascular and periadnexal infiltration of small to medium-sized cells with blastoid cytologic features is observed. In this patient, differentiation from skin involvement of mantle cell lymphoma was difficult in a section stained with haematoxylin and eosin although immunostaining could easily distinguish it.

- **Fig. 1:** Indurated erythematous plaque and papules on the face.
- **Fig. 2:** Dense nodular mononuclear cell infiltration around the vessels and adnexa (HE, microscopic magnification 10×).
- **Fig. 3:** Infiltration of small to medium-sized lymphoid cells. Small number of eosinophils are also present (HE; microscopic magnification 100×).
- **Fig. 4:** Most of the infiltrating cells are T cells (CD3 immunostaining; microscopic magnification 10×).
- **Fig. 5:** A few B cells are present in the infiltrates (CD79a immunostaining; microscopic magnification 10×).
- **Fig. 6:** Cyclin D1 is not expressed on the infiltrating cells (cyclin D1 immunostaining; microscopic magnification 10×).

References

Davis MD, Perniciaro C, Dahl PR et al. (1998) Exaggerated arthropod-bite lesions in patients with chronic lymphocytic leukemia: a clinical, histopathologic, and immunopathologic study of eight patients. J Am Acad Dermatol 39:27–35

Barzilai A, Shapiro D, Goldberg I, et al. (1999) Insect bite-like reaction in patients with hematologic malignant neoplasms. Arch Dermatol 135:1503–1507

Sen F, Medeiros LJ, Lu D et al. (2002) Mantle cell lymphoma involving skin: cutaneous lesions may be the first manifestation of disease and tumors often have blastoid cytologic features. Am J Surg Pathol 26:1312–1318

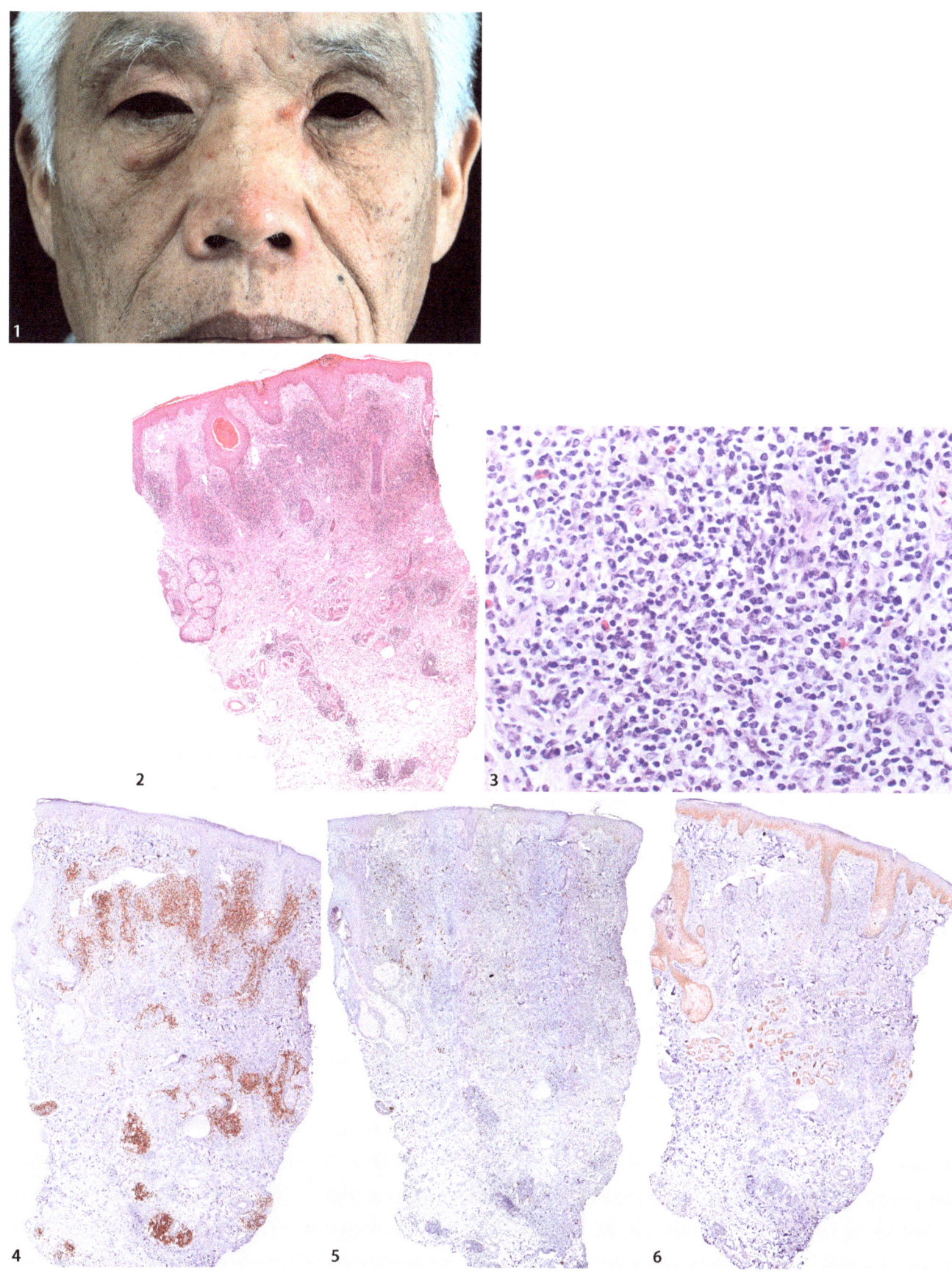

3 Immature Hematopoietic Malignancies

Blastic NK-cell lymphoma

H. Hashizume

Age: 75 years   **Sex:** M

Clinical features: Asymptomatic, red to purple nodules abruptly appeared and distributed on his scalp, body and knees in a month. Physical examinations showed cervical and axillar lymphadenopathy and hepatomagaly. Laboratory investigations revealed an increase in a peripheral white blood cell count (29700/µl with 14% of blast cells) and serum lactate dehydrogenase level (707 IU/l, normal 105–200 IU/l). An Epstein-Barr virus genome was not detected in the blood by the PCR method. T-cell receptor chain and immunoglobulin heavy chain were in germ configurations by Southern blot analysis of DNA extracted from the blood and the lesional skins. Bone marrow aspiration disclosed 73% of blast cells with myelodysplasia. Skin histology indicated dense infiltration of large atypical cells, positive for CD56 and CD123, at upper dermis and hair follicles. Extravasation of erythrocytes was also observed. Circulating blast cells expressed CD56, CD123, CD45RA and CD4, but not CD3 or CD45RO.

Diagnosis: Blastic NK-cell lymphoma (plasmacytoid DC leukaemia/lymphoma).

Follow-up: Combination chemotherapy with vincristine, pirarubicin, cyclophosphamide prednisolone and etoposide was partially effective for resolution of skin lesions and circulating blastic cells, but not bone marrow involvement. Six months after the therapy the eruption reappeared on the face with simultaneous emergence of circulating blastic cells. Secondary line chemotherapy will be considered.

Comment: Blastic NK cell lymphoma is a misnomer since the origin is now proven as the leukemic counterpart of plasmacytoid DC (Chaperot et al. 2001). Cutaneous lesions are frequently found as the first symptom corresponding to high expression of cutaneous lymphocyte antigen (CLA) in the blastoid cells (Petra et al. 2004). Final diagnosis depends on the expressions of CD4, CD56, CD123 (IL-3 receptor) and CD45RA, but not CD116 or CD45RO, in the blastic cells (Trimoreau et al.). Whereas most patients are initially sensitive to chemotherapy,

rapid relapse is common resulting in poor prognosis (Jacob et al. 2003). The blastic cells may dampen anti-tumor immune responses by promoting differentiation of naïve Th cells to Th2 cells (Chaperot et al. 2001).

- **Fig. 1:** Purple nodules on the trunk.
- **Fig. 2:** Dense infiltration of atypical cells in the dermis. HE, microscopic magnification $40\times$ (**a**) and $400\times$ (**b**).
- **Fig. 3:** CD56 (**a**) and CD123 (**b**) expressions of the infiltrating cells. Immunohistochemical staining, original microscopic magnification $200\times$.
- **Fig. 4:** Large cells (left, surrounded with red line) expressed CD4 (middle upper) and CD56 (middle lower), but not CD3. These cells were strongly positive for CD123 (right, upper) and HLA-DR (right, lower) by flow cytometric analysis. Numbers indicate percentages of the gated cells.
- **Fig. 5:** Purified circulating blast cells promoted Th2 cell differentiation of naïve allogeneic Th cells in vitro. Allogeneic CD4+CD45RO− cells co-cultured with CD56+ cells purified from the patient's peripheral blood cells for 4 days followed by expansion with IL-2, and re-stimulated with PMA and calcium ionophore for 24 h. Percentages of IL-4- and IFN-γ-producing cells were analyzed by flow cytometric analysis after intracytoplasmic cytokine staining. Numbers indicate percentages of total cells. Left, isotype control.

References

Chaperot L, Bendriss N, Manches O et al. (2001) Identification of a leukemic counterpart of the plasmacytoid dendritic cells. Blood 97:3210–3217

Jacob MC, Chaperot L, Mossuz P et al. (2003) CD4+ CD56+ lineage negative malignancies: a new entity developed from malignant early plasmacytoid dendritic cells. Haematologica 88:941–955

Petrella T, Meijer CJ, Dalac S et al. (2004) TCL1 and CLA expression in agranular CD4/CD56 hematodermic neoplasms (blastic NK-cell lymphomas) and leukemia cutis. Am J Clin Pathol 122:307–313

Trimoreau F, Donnard M, Turlure P et al. (2003) The CD4+ CD56+ CD116- CD123+CD45RA+ CD45RO- profile is specific of DC2 malignancies. Haematologica 88:ELT10

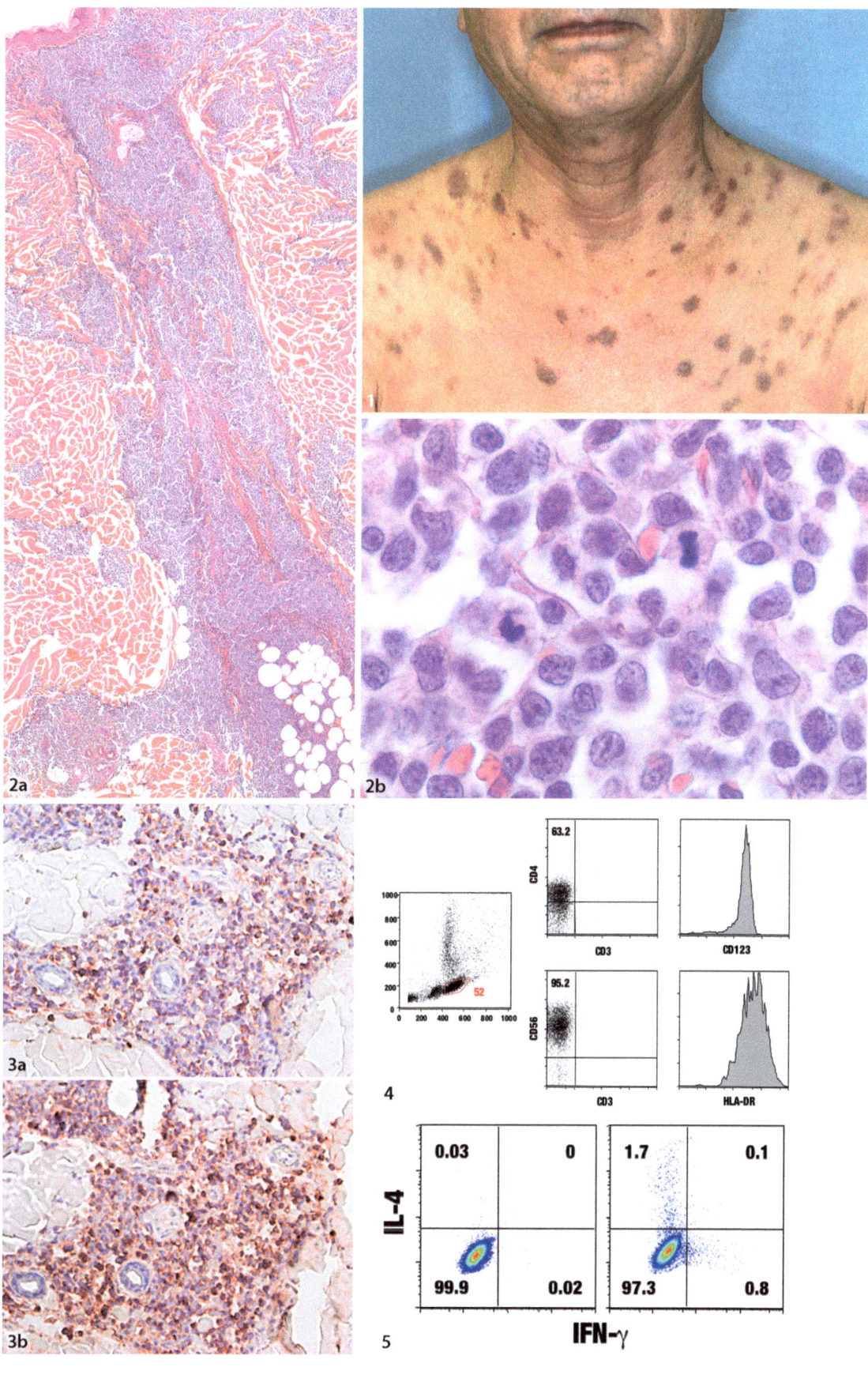

Subcutaneous splenosis of the abdominal wall

L. BOUDOVA, D. V. KAZAKOV, P. MUKENŠNABL, O. HES and M. MICHAL

Age: 23 years   **Sex:** M

Clinical features: An oligophrenic non-communicating inmate of a mental hospital was referred to a surgery department because of a subcutaneous mass in the abdominal wall. Clinical examination revealed an 8×7-cm, well-demarcated subcutaneous tumour in the left inguinal area closely above the scar after a previous operation for hernia. As no history could be taken from the patient, the provisional clinical diagnosis was a tumour of unknown origin or an incarcerated hernia. At operation, the tumour was confined to the subcutis, whereas the underlying abdominal fascia and muscles appeared intact. Grossly, the multinodular tumour was partially enveloped by thick fibrous bands. It was immobile, firmly embedded in the subcutaneous fat tissue. The dark red tumour measured 8×5×7 cm, and had a hard consistency. The cut surface revealed black hemorrhagic areas and a few irregular small whitish foci.

Diagnosis: Subcutaneous splenosis.

Comment: Splenosis is also referred to as autotransplantation of splenic tissue. It is represented by implants of splenic tissue in the form of encapsulated nodules localized typically on the peritoneal surface, while extraperitoneal sites including the subcutis are involved only very rarely. Splenosis follows a traumatic rupture of the spleen or surgery. In most cases, the pathogenesis is probably through mechanical implant, yet in the single published instance of cerebral splenosis, a hematogenous spread of splenic tissue is assumed. The interval between the splenic injury and the diagnosis is sometimes as long as several decades. In our case the causal event could not be identified in the patient's history due to his severe mental handicap.

Histologically, some cases of splenosis may be poorly developed architecturally and thus present a diagnostic challenge, as the microscopic picture may simulate a lymphoproliferative disorder. In other instances, a full complement of red and white pulp is readily recognizable, resulting in an appearance similar to that of accessory spleen. The latter would be the main differential diagnosis on solely microscopic grounds. However, the localization in the subcutis excludes the possibility of an accessory spleen which occurs in the tail of the pancreas or within the gastrosplenic ligament, reflecting the prenatal development of the abdominal viscera.

- **Fig. 1:** A formol-fixed specimen consists of multiple brown nodules of variable size embedded in subcutaneous fat. They are speckled with black haemorrhagic areas and small white infarcts.
- **Fig. 2:** A scanning magnification of a part of the lesion. Red pulp and follicles of white pulp are visible (HE).
- **Fig. 3:** An isolated subcutaneous nodule composed exclusively of congested red pulp might pose a diagnostic problem (HE).
- **Fig. 4:** Well-developed splenic structures: red pulp of cords of Billroth and slightly congested venous sinuses, and white pulp showing central arteries with periarteriolar lymphoid sheaths, follicles and marginal zones (HE, **a**); germinal centres are seen in some lymphoid follicles (HE, **b**).

References

Baack BR, Varsa EW, Burgdorf WH et al. (1990) Splenosis. A report of subcutaneous involvement. Am J Dermatopathol 12:585–588

Boudova L, Kazakov DV, Hes O, Zahálka M, Mukensnabl P, Kocová J, Michal M (2005) Subcutaneous splenosis of the abdominal wall. American Journal of Dermatopathology, accepted for publication, Aug 2005

Carr NJ, Turk EP (1992) The histological features of splenosis. Histopathology 21:549–553

Khosravi MR, Margulies DR, Alsabeh R, et al. (2004) Consider the diagnosis of splenosis for soft tissue masses long after any splenic injury. Am Surg 70:967–970

Rosai J (2004) Spleen, p. 2020. In: Rosai and Ackerman's Surgical Pathology, 9th edition. Mosby, Elsevier Inc. Vol 2. 2977 pages

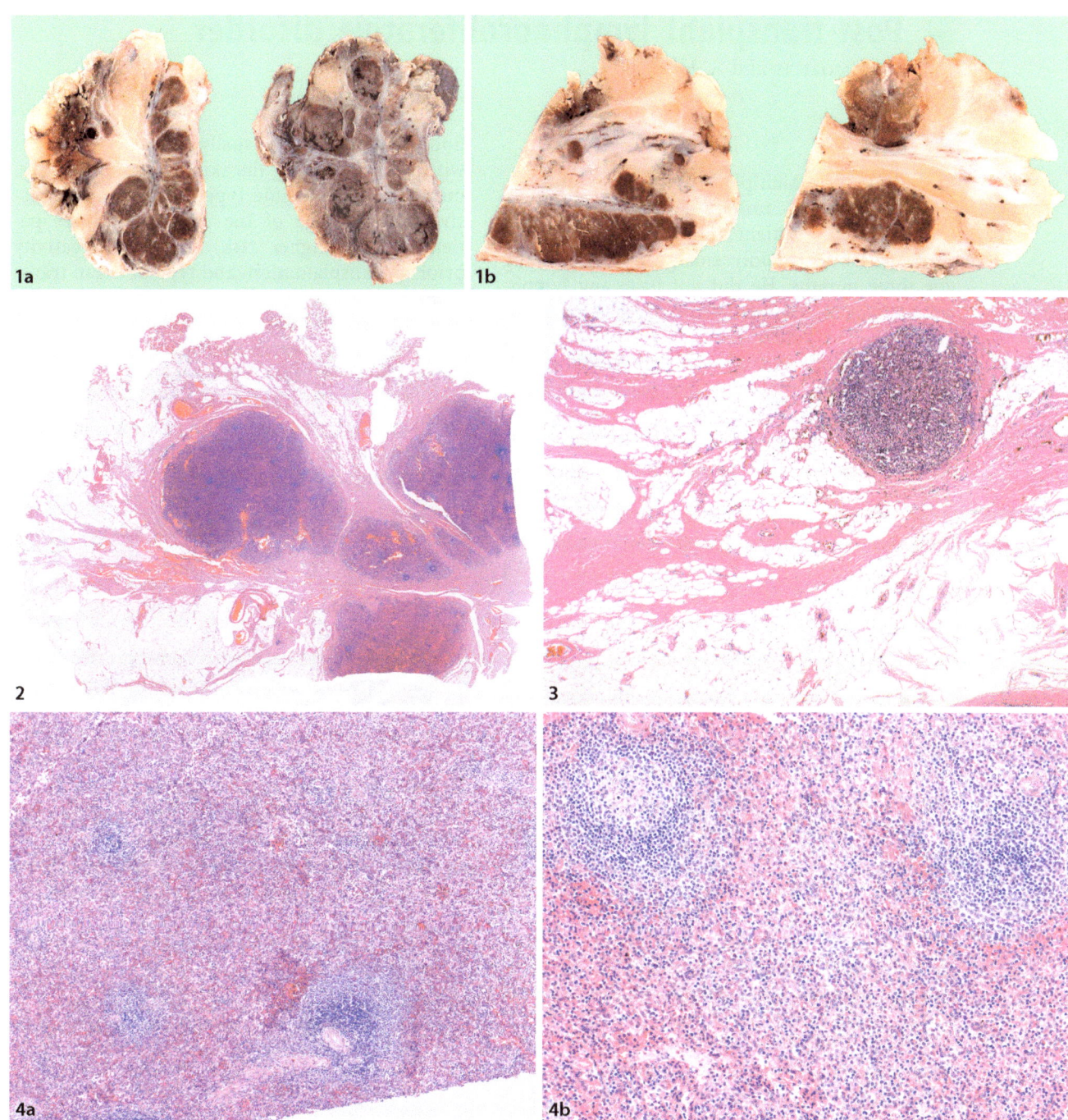

Post-transplant lymphoproliferative disorder

N. Samolitis and R. Harris

Age: 63 years   **Sex:** M

Clinical features: Multiple erythematous and necrotic exophytic tumors were observed in groups on the patient's right lower extremity. They had been rapidly enlarging and bleeding for three months. He did not have any lymphadenopathy in the involved extremity or inguinal area. The patient had a history of a cardiac transplant and was on multiple immunosuppressive agents. An extensive workup did not reveal evidence of lymphoma or myeloma involving any other organs. A skin biopsy revealed a dermal tumor consisting of atypical appearing lymphocytes with some plasmacytoid features. Immunohistochemical staining for CD138 confirmed the plasma cell lineage. In-situ hybridization for Epstein-Barr virus (EBV) was positive in the tumor cells.

Diagnosis: Post-transplant lymphoproliferative disorder (PTLD), plasmacytoid type.

Follow-up: The patient's immunosuppressive regimen was decreased and the localized area with tumor involvement was treated with superficial electron beam radiation. The tumors resolved and did not recur within 9 months of follow up, but the patient subsequently died from cardiac failure.

Comment: PTLD is a well-recognized complication of solid organ and bone marrow transplantation with immunosuppression. It is usually secondary to uncontrolled proliferation of EBV infected B-cells although some tumors (<10%) do not show evidence of EBV infection. PTLD has a variety of clinical manifestations ranging from a mononucleosis-type illness (polyclonal form) to lymphoma (monoclonal form). It usually presents in the GI tract, liver, lymph nodes, kidney, lung or in the transplanted organ. PTLD is rarely seen in the skin and underlying organ or lymph node involvement is usually present in patients with PTLD involving the skin. Risks for development of PTLD include type of immunosuppressive regimen, age of the patient (younger patients are at higher risk), EBV seronegativity prior to transplantation, and type of organ transplanted (cardiac transplant patients are at the highest risk). In mild cases, decreasing immunosuppression is usually adequate treatment. In more advanced cases, chemotherapy and radiation may be necessary. Rituxamab, an anti-CD20 antibody, may be useful in tumors expressing predominantly CD20 positive B-cells (the most common type of PTLD).

Fig. 1: Multiple erythematous, necrotic papules and exophytic tumors on the lower extremity.

Fig. 2: Nodular dermal tumor. HE, microscopic magnification 20×.

Fig. 3: Atypical cells with some plasmacytoid features and mitotic activity. HE, microscopic magnification 200×.

Fig. 4: Intense staining for the plasma cell marker CD138. Microscopic magnification 200×. Inset with high magnification.

Fig. 5: Lack of staining for the B-cell marker CD20. Microscopic magnification 200×.

Fig. 6: Kappa restriction, indicating monoclonality. Microscopic magnification 200×.

References

Samolitis NJ, Bharadwaj JS, Weis JR, Harris RM et al. (2004) Post-transplant lymphoproliferative disorder limited to the skin. J Cutan Pathol 31:453–457

Nalesnik MA (2001) The diverse pathology of post-transplant lymphoproliferative disorders: the importance of a standardized approach. Transpl Infect Dis 3:88–96

Schumann KW, Oriba HA, Bergfeld WF et al. (2000) Cutaneous presentation of posttransplant lymphoproliferative disorder. J Am Acad Dermatol 42:923–926

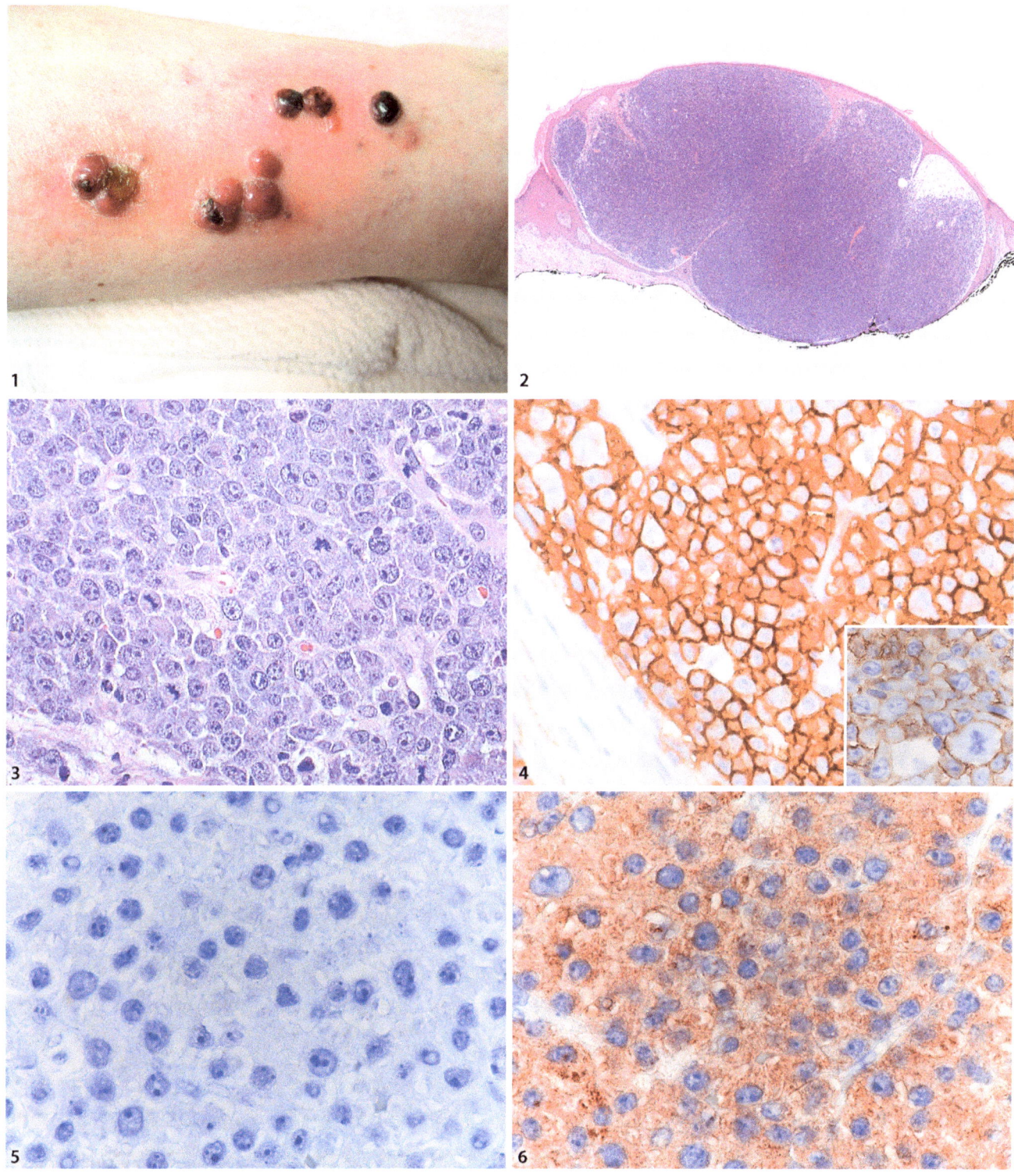

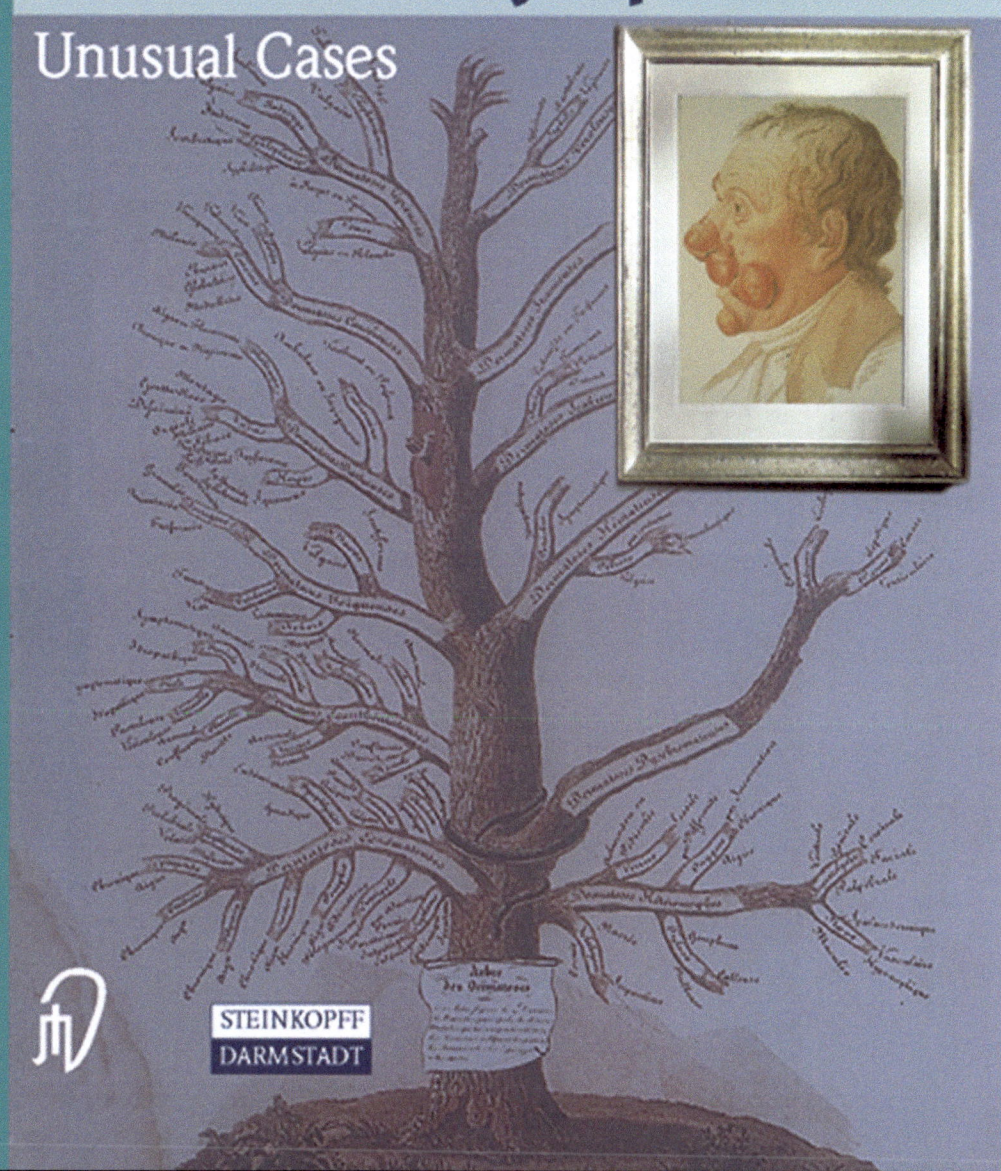

GÜNTER BURG · PHILIP E. LEBOIT
Editors

WERNER KEMPF · BEATRIX MÜLLER
Co-Editors

Cutaneous Lymphomas

Unusual Cases

STEINKOPFF
DARMSTADT

2001 · 107 pp · 328 col. fig. · Hardcover · EUR 99,95* · ISBN 3-7985-1250-7
*Prices are net-prices subject to local VAT

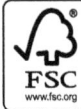

MIX
Papier aus verantwortungsvollen Quellen
Paper from responsible sources
FSC® C105338

If you have any concerns about our products,
you can contact us on
ProductSafety@springernature.com

In case Publisher is established outside the EU,
the EU authorized representative is:
Springer Nature Customer Service Center GmbH
Europaplatz 3, 69115 Heidelberg, Germany

Printed by Libri Plureos GmbH
in Hamburg, Germany